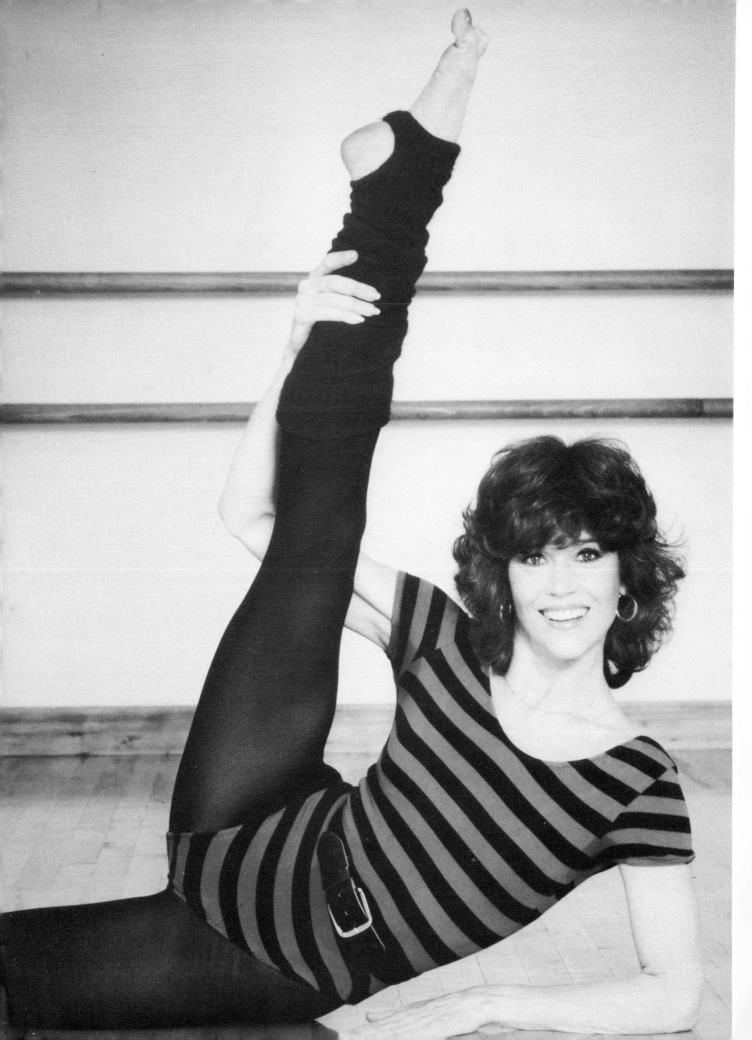

Jane Fonda's Workout Book

by Jane Fonda

Photographs by Steve Schapiro

Allen Lane

ALLEN LANE
Penguin Books Ltd
536 Kings road
London SW10 0UH

First published in the U.S.A. by Simon & Schuster 1981
First published in Great Britain by Allen Lane 1982

Reprinted 1982 (six times)
Reprinted 1983 (three times)

ISBN 0 7139 1437 8

Printed in Great Britain by
Butler & Tanner Ltd
Frome and London

Designed by Eve Metz
Photo Editor—Vincent Virga

The author is grateful to Crown Publishers, Inc.,
for permission to reprint menu on page 233
from *Eat Your Heart Out* by Jim Hightower,
copyright © 1975 by Jim Hightower.

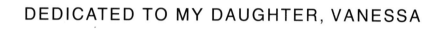
DEDICATED TO MY DAUGHTER, VANESSA

ACKNOWLEDGEMENTS

My special thanks to the following friends who have given their support and expertise:

Mary Kushner, Paul Blanc, Dr. Michael Jacobson, Carol Gutierrez, Lesley Mallgrave, Karen Nussbaum, David White, Steve Kelly, Vincent Virga, Nan Talese, Judy Kaplan, Barbara Wyden, my favorite photographer Steve Schapiro, his assistant Steve Shaffer, and Leni Cazden, wherever you are.

Contents

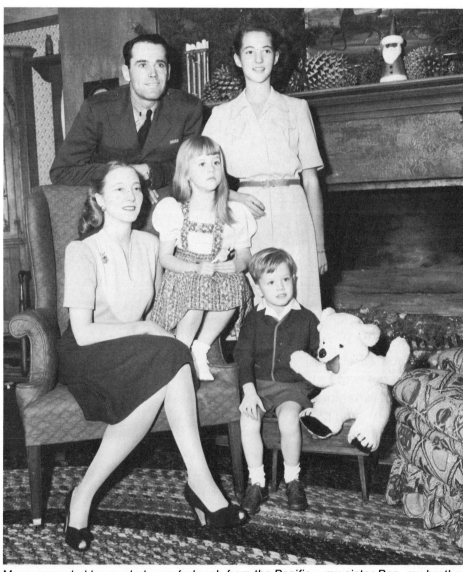

Me, surrounded by my dad—on furlough from the Pacific—my sister Pan, my brother Peter, and my mother, Frances

Prologue

Like a great many women, I am a product of a culture that says thin is better, blond is beautiful and buxom is best.

From as early as I can remember, my mother, her friends, my grandmother, governesses, my sister—all the women who surrounded me—talked anxiously about the pros and cons of their physiques. Hefty thighs, small breasts, a biggish bottom—there was always some perceived imperfection to focus anxieties on. None of them seemed happy the way they were, which bewildered me because the way they were seemed fine to my young eyes.

In pursuit of the "feminine ideal"—exemplified by voluptuous film stars and skinny fashion models—women, it seemed, were even prepared to do violence to themselves. My mother, for example, who was a rather slender, beautiful woman, was terrified of getting fat. She once said that if she ever gained weight she'd have the excess flesh cut off! I remember a friend of hers talking about being injected with the urine of pregnant cows, which was reputed to make fat dissolve.

Maybe I simply wasn't privy to their more intimate conversations, but I don't remember the men in my life being as concerned about how they looked. Not with the same angst at any rate. If anything, they seemed more interested in performance: making the team, doing the job, being brave. The message that came across was clear: men were judged by their accomplishments, women by their looks.

Like many young girls, I internalized this message and, in an effort to conform to the sought-after female image, I abused my health, starved my body, and ingested heaven-knows-what chemical drugs. I understood very little about how my body functioned, and what it needed to be healthy and strong. I depended on doctors to cure me, but never relied on myself to stay well.

It wasn't until I was thirty, and pregnant for the first time, that I began to change the way I treated myself. As the baby grew inside me, I began to realize my body needed to be listened to and strengthened, not ignored and weakened. I discovered that with common sense, a bit of studying and a good deal of commitment, I could create for myself a new approach to health and beauty: an approach which would not only make me look better, but would enable me to handle the intense, multi-faceted life I live with more clarity and balance, to say nothing of more energy and endurance.

I decided to write this book, not because I consider myself an expert in the pedigreed sense, but because I want to share what I've had to learn the hard way with other women. I only wish someone had shared these things with me earlier in my life. That's why I've dedicated this book to my daughter.

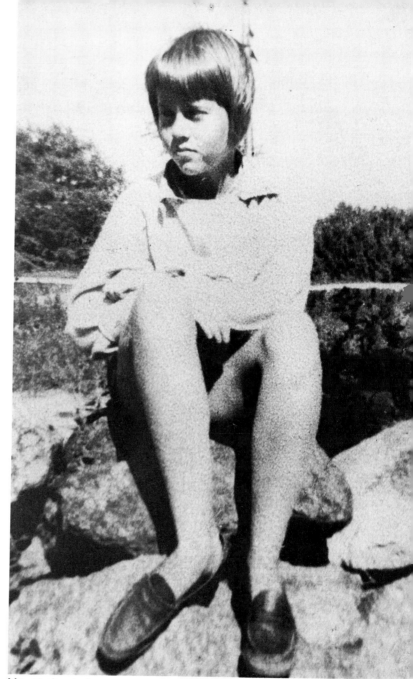
Me, at about eleven

Part One
Lessons Learned

A Body Abused

As a child, I was your basic klutz—awkward, plump and self-conscious. I was convinced that when God passed out gracefulness, I had dropped my share. I could hardly get across a room without bumping into something. I resented my body. I felt that a different, more interesting me had been imprisoned in the wrong body. Somehow I had been betrayed.

Objectively, things probably were not all that bad. My father and mother thought I was adorable. It was not as if people would look at me and whisper, ''Oh, my God, look at that fat little girl!'' What is important, though, is how I perceived myself. I felt plump and clumsy and so I behaved plump and clumsy.

Psychologists have learned that people's perception of themselves is much more powerful in determining personality and behavior than the way they actually look. I know beautiful women who consider themselves homely because when they were young their striking features set them apart. I also know women who are far from beautiful in the classic sense, but who take your breath away because they exude such an air of confidence in themselves and their looks that we perceive them as beautiful. And I know thin women who think of themselves as fat, because they were fat when they were young. I was so conditioned to thinking of myself as fat that later, when I was really thin, I could never convince myself that I was thin enough.

If anyone had told me when I was a teenager that the time would come when I would run several miles a day and work out until I was dripping with sweat, I would have thought he was crazy. I never enjoyed sports. I was uncoordinated and had little endurance. I had athletic friends who kicked and dribbled, jumped and ran with seeming effortlessness, but I had no desire to join them. In fact, I welcomed the occasional earache or cramps that gave me an excuse to skip phys. ed. I liked to swim and I was a good rider, but that was the extent of my athletic abilities and interest.

When I was fourteen, I went to a girls' boarding school. It was there that my friends and I developed a preoccupation with food. Eating binges were *de rigueur*. In retrospect, I suppose this was a way of relieving boredom and our budding sexual tensions. I remember bingeing on coffee ice cream by the gallon and pound cake by the pound. We

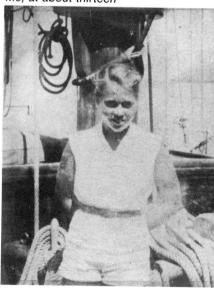

Me, at about thirteen

bought bagfuls of brownies and gobbled them down. We stuffed ourselves with peanut butter and bacon sandwiches. These food binges continued right through my years at Vassar, interspersed with crash diets as I frantically tried to get slimmed down and pulled together for the occasional dance or weekend away.

In my freshman year at boarding school, we discovered advertisements in our hidden cache of *True Confessions* magazines telling us that by sending money and a coupon we would receive chewing gum that would make us lose weight. My roommate believed (I don't know if she was right) that it was because the gum contained tapeworm eggs which would hatch inside us. We presumed that the food we ate would be devoured by the tapeworm before it was absorbed by us. Sharing life with a tapeworm seemed a small price to pay for thinness. We dutifully sent in our coupons and chewed the gum, but it didn't work. Maybe the eggs were dead. What a rip-off, we thought.

Our binges sometimes progressed to revolting extremes. I remember one year when we studied Roman civilization, we came across a footnote explaining how the Romans made a practice of retreating to a room known as the vomitorium during their orgiastic feasts. After inducing vomiting, they would return to the feast and start all over again.

"Ah-ha," we thought, "here's a way to *not* have our cake and eat it too!" We could indulge our compulsions without having to face the consequences of getting fat. It gave us a heady sense of being in control. I had absolutely no idea that I was establishing an indulgence/deprivation cycle that would become psychologically and physically addictive. The more we vomited ourselves into emptiness, the more we needed to eat. I didn't understand for a long time that the act of vomiting causes a sudden drop in blood sugar which, in turn, produces a craving for more food. And so it would begin all over again leaving us, ultimately, weakened and depressed. This binge-and-vomit cycle, known as bulimarexia, is most prevalent among pre-adolescent and adolescent girls. I think it may be caused in large part by the combination of the social pressure to be thin and an almost infantile need to prove that you can be in control at least of your own body, if nothing else.

Our school never provided any counseling on health and nutrition except for the tedious general science course we had to take, and nothing we learned in this course seemed to apply to our own lives. We probably would not have paid attention even if it had. Our obsession with eating and dieting was more important than any consideration of good nutrition or basic good health. We felt immortal. We took health for granted.

At Vassar, I discovered Dexedrine. We called them pep pills; today they are called speed. When we were cramming for exams, or staying up all night finishing our term papers, the pills kept us alert and awake. We soon discovered that taking Dexedrine had what we considered a splendid side effect. It took away our appetites. So we began taking the pills to lose weight. We never once had difficulty in finding a doctor to write a prescription. No doctor ever took the time, or showed enough interest, to ask us just how and why we were using these amphetamines. Nor did any doctor ever warn us that we could become addicted to them—as I did. I used them—needing more and more as time went by to get the same effect—and didn't stop until I realized that I was losing control of my life. But it was not easy. There is a terrible sense of fatigue and depression when you stop after using pills for years.

When I left Vassar, I enrolled in the Actors Studio in New York City where I studied under Lee Strasberg. Since I wanted to be independent, I worked as a model to pay my tuition. Frankly, I was astonished at the success I had as a model. Within a few months I was on the covers of *Vogue, Glamour, Esquire,* and *Parade.* Although my body had lost its adolescent plumpness, I still thought of myself as fat and worried constantly about losing weight. I lived on (wince) cigarettes, coffee, speed and strawberry yogurt.

But try as I might, I just couldn't seem to lose the round-cheeked all-American girl-next-door look. It seemed so boring. What I yearned for was to look like Suzy Parker, the top model of the day, whose hollow-cheeked angularity seemed the pinnacle of beauty.

I was thin now, but with those cheeks, I would never fit into the Suzy Parker mold of beauty. Still, I was determined to.

In boarding school, I had discovered vomiting, in college Dexedrine, and as a model I learned about diuretics. A number of my friends went to a doctor who, they said, could make you lose weight. What he did was write you a prescription for a diuretic, a little white pill that you

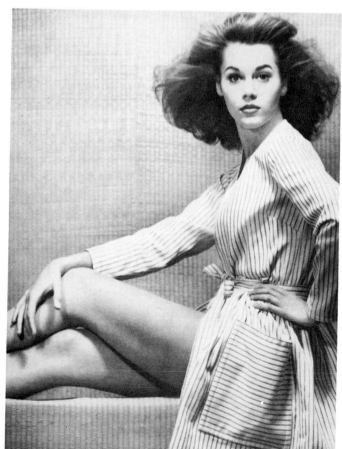

As a fashion model, 1960

were supposed to take once every three days. Diuretics ''shrink'' your body by forcing the fluids out. The results were just what I wanted. Inches seemed to evaporate overnight.

I took diuretics for almost twenty years, almost half my lifetime, something that appalls me today. I had to keep increasing the dosage, because the longer I took them, the less effective they were. By the time I was in my late thirties, I was taking two or three a day. I had no idea of what I was doing to myself. These pills turned what had been a really minor problem of fluid retention into a chronic one.

No doctor—and there were many through the years who gave me prescriptions for diuretics and stimulants—ever told me of their side effects or advised me to take potassium to make up for the potassium that I was losing. When the body level of potassium is low, it can cause severe muscle weakness, fatigue and depression. The most serious side effect of prolonged use of diuretics is that it can cause the kidneys to lose their ability to concentrate urine. This results in frequent urination and causes serious losses of the water-soluble B vitamins.

Anyone who absolutely must be on diuretics should make sure she has a good source of potassium in her diet. Bananas and citrus fruit are probably the best, but melons, dried fruits, beans and potatoes also have abundant potassium. And you should take a vitamin B_6 supplement every day, approximately 60 milligrams, to help replace the vitamin excreted in the urine.

I did not stop taking diuretics until 1976 when I was in London making *Julia* and was fortunate enough to meet a wonderful naturopathic doctor, whose holistic approach to health combined acupuncture, natural medicine, chiropractic and nutrition. Rarities in this country, these doctors abound in England and France. He explained to me how my prolonged use of diuretics had weakened my kidneys and told me about safer natural diuretics such as parsley juice. He treated me with acupuncture and gave me a homeopathic remedy for fluid retention. I have not taken a chemical diuretic since. I still have a tendency to retain fluid, but I find I can control it with strenuous exercise and an occasional herbal diuretic.

Until I met this doctor, no one had ever explained that there were other ways of losing weight besides starvation diets, Dexedrine and diuretics, ways that would not damage my body. As a matter of fact, no doctor had ever told me that I was damaging my body with all this chemical tinkering. Looking back, I realize that to a large extent I was a victim of medical malpractice.

If I had only known what I was doing to myself! If I had only understood twenty years ago the futility, the alienation, the self-denigration of trying to fit oneself into a mold. It was as if I was thinking of myself as a product rather than a person. I had yet to learn that the most incredible beauty and the most satisfying way of life come from affirming your own uniqueness, making the most of what you really are. The glow and energy of the healthy woman is the ultimate beauty, the only beauty that will last.

We Become What We Do

I will never forget the day in 1959 when I was made up for my first movie, *Tall Story,* in which I played a cheerleader and my costar, Tony Perkins, played a college basketball star. I was tilted back in what looked like a dentist's chair in the makeup department of Warner Brothers for hours while the makeup men and hair stylists worked on me.

When they were through, I could hardly recognize myself in the mirror—winged eyebrows, false eyelashes, big pink lips, hair that looked as if it had been ironed, right off the Warner Brothers assembly line together with Sandra Dee, Connie Stevens, Dorothy Provine, and others. But these men were experts with awesome reputations and I was just a model from New York. A lot of time and effort and money were being spent to make me a star. Who was I to claim to understand the mysteries of the motion picture camera? They were the professionals; they must know what they were doing.

The anxious concern that my mother and her friends had devoted to their faces and bodies when I was a child was nothing to what confronted me now. During my first few weeks in Hollywood, I was told that Jack Warner, the head of the studio, did not believe that a small-breasted woman could become a star. And shortly after that at some party or other, a prominent film director suggested that I seriously consider having my back teeth pulled and my jaw broken. He told me that another baby-faced actress in search of cheekbones had had this done successfully. I spent a good part of the next dozen years as a blonde, with false eyelashes and false breasts, and while my jaw remained intact, my spirit didn't.

The Hollywood emphasis on looks filled me with anxiety. Despite my modeling, I had always felt that if I had anything special to offer, it was not my looks. I used to walk down the street in those early days feeling that the real me was someplace else, that the present occupant of my body, the "she" that was Jane Fonda, was someone I was not sure I knew—or liked.

I yearned to recapture the excitement I had felt as a student at the Actors Studio—the challenge of plumbing the depths of a complex woman character until I not only understood her, but was able to find her essence within myself. I chafed under the constraints of the ingenue roles I was asked to play which required only that I be cute. There were

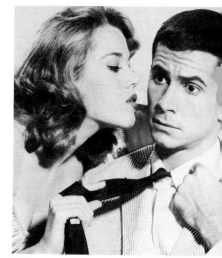

With Tony Perkins in Tall Story

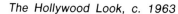

The Hollywood Look, c. 1963

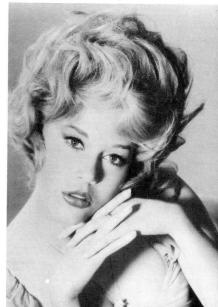

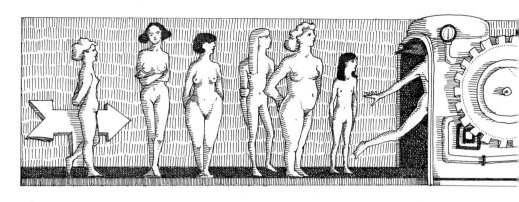

no challenges, no opportunities to extend myself. But I felt unable to change the situation.

What I did not realize was that the situation was changing me. Year after year, movie after movie, the characters I was playing were little bitty, one-dimensional girls, and this had its effect on me. After a while I stopped rebelling against my glossy vacuous roles. The deeper, more complex and exciting parts of me began to atrophy from lack of use. I was becoming more and more like my characters.

I have spent a lot of time thinking about this part of my life and observing how work affects people's lives. I am convinced that we become what we do. If our work is stimulating and rewarding, if it pushes us to grow in understanding and knowledge, we become more valuable human beings and relish not only our work, but the other facets of our lives. But if our work is belittling and stressful, if it provides little or no fulfillment, offers no sense of participation, this can have a negative effect. In time, our full human potential will simply shrivel up and we may not even be aware that it is happening. I certainly had not been.

I learned to fit into Hollywood. I became a successful movie star. And with the movie *Barbarella,* my image as a sex symbol was established. *Barbarella,* based on a French comic book character, was the first sexy, camp, science fiction-adventure film. In the titles, I appeared floating naked in space, and after that in an array of bizarre and revealing outfits. As Barbarella, I overcame everything, because Barbarella's sexual potency was so dynamic that it destroyed everything that stood in her way. Now that I look back on it, as a sex fantasy it had a certain charm and freshness. But as I said, it stamped me as a sex symbol.

A feminist asked me in 1969 how I had felt doing *Barbarella.* "It must have done strange things to you," she said. I went absolutely blank. I did not know how to answer her, because I did not understand what she meant. I did not know she was referring to the personal cost of being turned into a sexual object. I did not even realize that I had been. The burgeoning new women's consciousness had not yet found its way into my mind and heart.

My only thought was that no one had forced me to make the film. If I starved, dyed and painted myself into that role, it was my own doing. I was completely unaware of the extent to which I had internalized the cultural pressures that associate a woman's success with sex and a surface kind of beauty until several years later, when it struck me under circumstances that were as far removed from *Barbarella* as this galaxy is from the next.

It was the spring of 1972 and I had just met my future husband, Tom

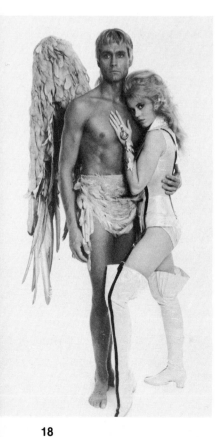

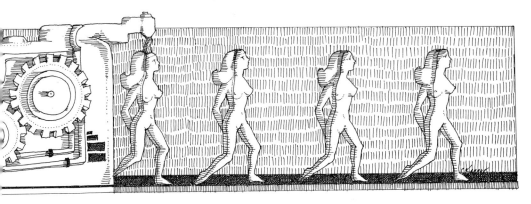

Hayden. Both of us were activists in the movement against the war in Vietnam. I had put together a slide show on Vietnam and was showing it in union halls, churches and for community groups. It concentrated almost entirely on the damage that we were doing with our bombing of Indochina. Tom had also put together a slide show. He had seen mine and one day he called and we arranged to get together so he could show me his. I think he wanted me to see it so that I could understand how the impact of destruction is only truly felt when you realize what it is that you are destroying.

His presentation began with an unusually beautiful series of slides showing the history and culture of the Vietnamese, a people who had lived in harmony with the land and whose most hallowed institution was the family. It described the centuries-old life of the villages, the economic interdependence and the common struggle against natural calamities and outside invaders that bound village to village.

Tom's slides showed how the elderly were respected. I remember one photograph in particular, a grinning leathery-faced grandmother holding a baby on her hip. She had that vital dignity that comes from having a valued and respected role in the family and the community. The elderly were not only needed to help tend the children, they passed along the accumulated wisdom of their life experiences to the younger generations. When they died, they were buried in the rice fields surrounding the village. Generation after generation lived in the presence of their ancestors' graves, the bones of the past fertilizing the rice which feeds the future, an eternal natural cycle, whole and complete. The Vietnamese believe that if a body is not buried, the spirit cannot rest. When the villages and rice fields were bombed, the ancestral graves were annihilated, leaving the spirits to wander homeless.

Along with the bombing, there was a program called Forced Urbanization. Families were broken up, destroying the delicate fabric of Vietnamese village society. Hundreds of thousands of peasants from the villages were herded into the crowded cities, all of which had heartbreakingly high rates of unemployment. There was no work for the peasants. In order to survive, the men became soldiers and, in desperation, many young village women became prostitutes.

The slides portrayed the lives of a modest people who were profoundly influenced by Buddhism, and who shared the Buddhist concept of the perfect human body as the innocent form of a little girl. And then Tom showed one slide that I will never forget. It was of a huge billboard in Saigon showing a larger-than-life Asian woman in a Playboy Bunny type of pose. The billboard was advertising the services of an American plastic surgeon whose specialty was changing Vietnamese women's eyes from their natural almond shape to the rounder shape of the Caucasian eye. For a little more money, he also performed operations to enlarge breasts and buttocks. Apparently, a prostitute could increase her price with her American tricks if she conformed to the Western playboy sexual standard. And these operations weren't confined only to prostitutes. Many of them were done on women in ''high society'' such as the wives of Generals Thieu and Ky. These women, literally, had their faces and bodies Americanized.

As I thought about what this slide implied, I began to see my own life with new eyes. The women of Vietnam had become victims of the same *Playboy* culture that had played havoc with me. I had used pills and near-starvation diets rather than surgery, but we had both gone against our own natures and bodies to achieve an imposed ideal of beauty. God knows what it did to their minds. I know what it did to mine. I was shocked into the realization that I myself had played an unwitting role as a movie star and sex symbol in perpetrating the stereotypes that affected women all over the world.

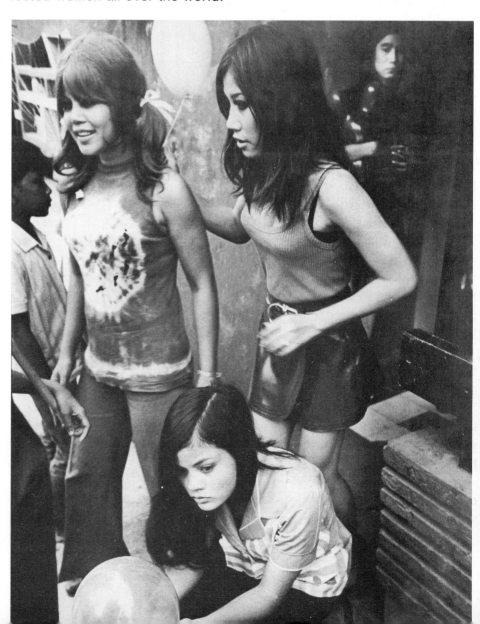

The Positive Approach

Despite all the abuse I showered on my body over the years, there was one positive thing I did. I studied ballet. How I started was completely accidental. I was in my early twenties, and my boyfriend was a dancer who taught jazz dancing at the June Taylor School in New York City. I enrolled in his classes mainly because I loved to watch him move, but my attention was drawn more and more to the ballet classes being taught next door. The ballet teacher, by the way, was Richard Thomas, father of actor Richard Thomas, star of the TV series, "The Waltons."

I began studying ballet with him and soon got hooked. It was the first type of strenuous physical activity that had ever interested me. I liked its rigor, its precision, and the demands it made on my body. As I progressed I felt much more confident about myself. I learned to control my body and feel graceful. Not that I was ever very good; actually I never got beyond the intermediate level, and pirouettes were the bane of my existence (still are). But I did a mean *barre*. Visitors to the class could have mistaken me for a professional dancer—as long as they left before we moved from the *barre* to center floor.

No matter where I had to go to make a film, my first order of business was always to find the best ballet teacher I could and start taking classes. A *plié* is called a *plié* whether you are in London or Rome or Leningrad. I had only to walk into a dance class to feel immediately at home no matter where I was. The universal language of dance became the connecting link in my nomadic actress' life. I cherished my hours in ballet class day after day, year after year.

Sometimes it would mean getting up at dawn to take a class. Other times my co-workers would wonder why at the end of a fourteen-hour day on a stuffy sound stage I pushed myself to drive to ballet school, instead of joining them in collapsing with a drink. I certainly felt more like collapsing than working and sweating until I ached, but afterwards I would feel alive and revitalized. It was hard to explain this or to describe how good I felt about being disciplined.

What I was discovering on my own was that the more good things I did for my body, the less I needed the bad things. After ballet class I would not even feel like eating or drinking before I went to bed. The more I practiced discipline in this one area, the more discipline I was able to exert on myself in others.

There were times, of course, when I was tempted to pack it in. It would have been so easy. But I played a sort of game with myself that helped. I pretended I was a professional dancer who had to go on stage and perform no matter what. *Had* to. There were no excuses. None at all. This little "pretend" really helped. And at times when everything else in my life seemed to be falling apart, ballet was the constant that ran through my life like a spinal cord, holding it all together, giving it consistency, pulling me through.

For the last few years, my Workout has replaced ballet as the constant in my life. I discovered the exhilaration and rewards of working out after I broke my foot while completing filming on *The China Syndrome,* in which I played a television news reporter covering a near-accident in a nuclear plant. Michael Douglas and I were running to get on a helicopter. I was wearing four-inch platform sandals and I stumbled and broke my foot. In two months' time I was supposed to put on a bikini and start filming *California Suite.* I panicked. I would have less than three weeks after they took the cast off my foot to get in shape. At forty, that is not a lot of time, especially when you have been practically immobile for five weeks, weighed down by a plaster cast. And I knew that my foot would not be strong enough when the cast came off for me to take ballet and get back into shape that way.

My stepmother, Shirlee Fonda, came to my rescue. She took me to an exercise class that put me through the most vigorous and thorough workout I had ever had. I was so sore for the next three days that even getting into a car was an ordeal. I went to this class for an hour-and-a-half workout every day, sometimes twice a day, and I got in shape in time for *California Suite.*

I had gone to exercise classes before and found them boring. They offered no challenge. They never made me sweat. The class that Shirlee introduced me to, taught by a remarkable woman named Leni Cazden, was different from anything I had ever experienced. I really knew that I had worked every single part of my body at the end of that class.

Late that fall, I went to Utah to make *The Electric Horseman,* and I found myself with no place to exercise. I am one of those people who finds it excruciatingly difficult to exercise by myself. There were no ballet classes and no exercise classes in St. George, Utah, but there was a small spa. I had never taught before, but I went over one morning and asked if it would be all right for me to teach an exercise class at the spa at night after work. I made it clear that they did not have to pay me for it—I was doing it for myself and anyone else who might be interested in coming to join me.

Word got out and the room filled up every night with men from the film crew, high school girls, young married women, middle-aged women. There was one woman over sixty years old who told me she had been on heavy medication for fifteen years. I watched that woman

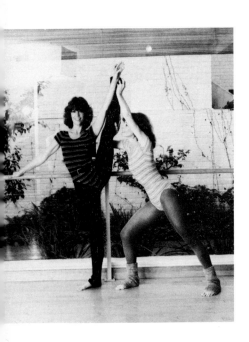

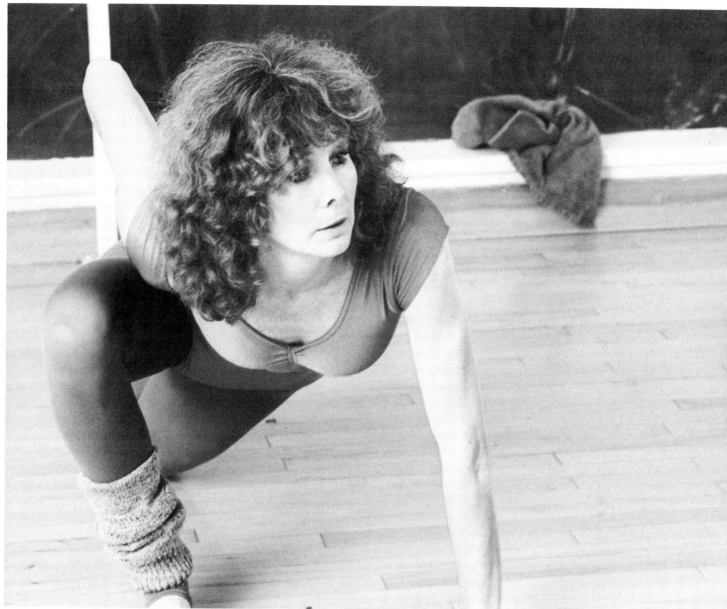

My stepmother, Shirlee Fonda

change as she came to work out night after night. After class one night she told me, "I haven't taken any medication for a week. It's the first time in fifteen years that I haven't had to take it."

I taught for six weeks and learned an enormous amount from these women by observing the effect that working out had on them. Some said it helped their menstrual cramps, others reported that they were losing weight, or losing inches. But most important, I discovered that working out had a definite effect on their attitudes about themselves. They felt better about themselves, held their heads higher and looked more comfortable in their bodies. I decided then that I wanted to offer the benefits of this kind of workout to more people. I opened my first Workout Studio about a year later.

Working out has become a part of my life. Almost anything else in my day can go by the board, but I must work out. If I didn't approach it that way, I probably could not do it at all, because there is always something that comes up. But I have made it a constant in my life.

As I had done earlier with ballet, when I approach my Workout I play a game of "pretend." I am no longer Jane Fonda, the actress, wife, mother, activist. I am an athlete. I *have* to push myself to my limit and beyond because I'm preparing for competition. But the competition is with myself. My commitment to working out has a lot to do with my high energy level. Today at forty-three my body is stronger and more limber, and I look and feel better, than when I was twenty.

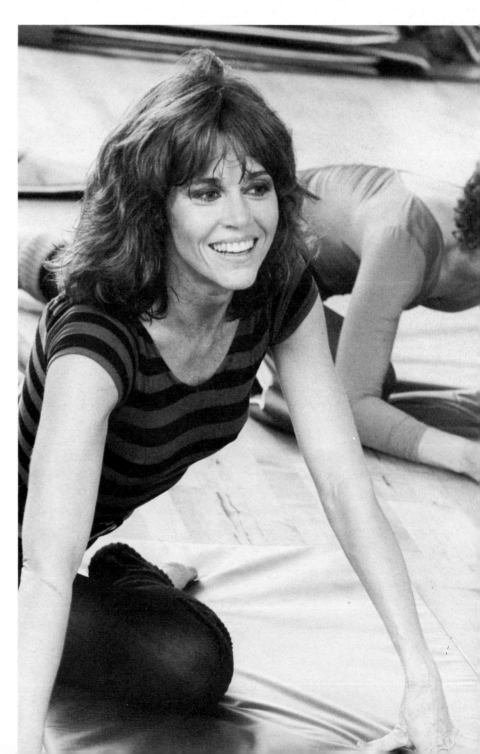

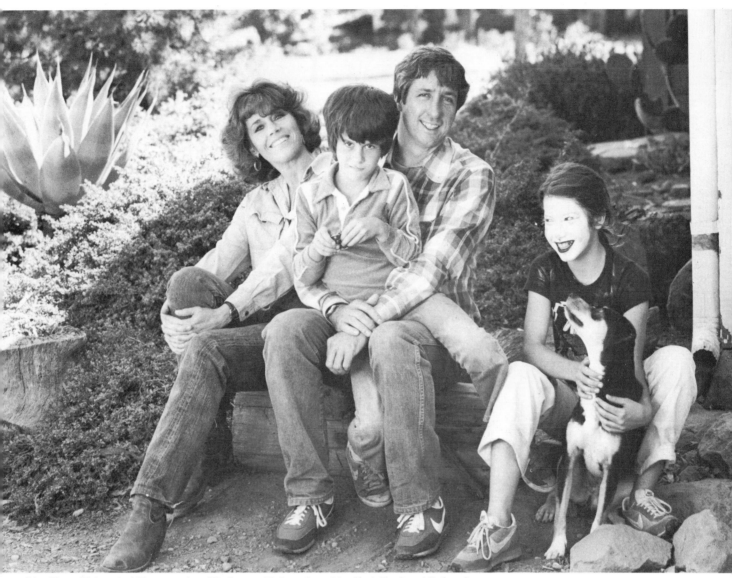

Me, Troy, Tom, and Vanessa in whiteface with her dog, Manila (also in whiteface)

Part Two
Wholly Health

Waking Up

Nutritionally

t is not only exercise that gives me energy and vitality. I have also earned to eat properly for health and beauty.

I was thirty when I became pregnant for the first time, and with pregnancy came something that I had never felt before—a sense of responsibility for my body. I had waited a long time to become pregnant; it was not as if I was in my late teens or twenties. I didn't know if I'd ever be pregnant again, and I wanted to do it right.

I became aware that I was going through the heaviest changes that I had experienced since adolescence. My body was literally telling me things. Sleep more. Eat better. I found myself drinking a lot of milk, something I had not done before. I no longer wanted to drink coffee. I had been a smoker, but while I was pregnant, the desire for cigarettes vanished. As I realized all this, I began consciously listening to what my body was telling me.

I felt that I was very alone—just me and my changing body. I yearned for a doctor who would give me advice on what to do in these crucial months so that my baby would be strong and healthy, but even in 1967 I couldn't find a doctor who was aware of the dangers that coffee, salt, cigarettes, and medicines presented to a pregnant woman and the child she was carrying. So I bought my first books on nutrition, and because I had no sympathetic doctor, I dogmatically followed their advice. Adelle Davis' book was my favorite. By the time I gave birth, it had fallen apart. I had read and reread every word of it, underlined it, studied it. It became my bible.

I wince when I think back on the day when, distraught, I went to a Beverly Hills pediatrician to ask why my four-month-old daughter Vanessa was not tolerating the bottle of goat's milk, dessicated baby veal liver, blackstrap molasses and cranberry juice concentrate I was giving her. I had nursed Vanessa for a month and a half and then I had started to wean her because I had to prepare for *They Shoot Horses, Don't They?*, which was scheduled to start in a couple of months. I had consulted my nutrition books and evolved what I thought was a health-giving meal for my baby. But Vanessa kept spitting it up. Who wouldn't?

That Beverly Hills pediatrician lifted an eyebrow and told me to forget about the goat's milk and the dessicated baby veal liver and all the rest and give Vanessa a baby formula called Similac. And that was that.

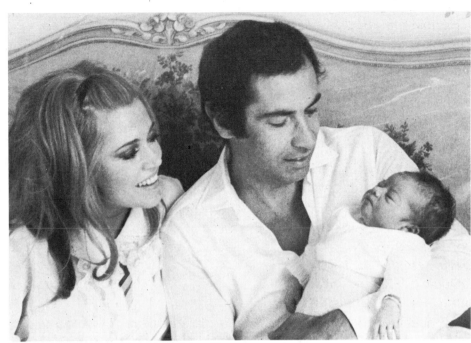

With Roger Vadim and our daughter, Vanessa

Had he been a doctor who was interested in the kind of approach I had to health, he would probably have sat down with me and explained why my little daughter could not tolerate the bottles I prepared for her. I was giving her too rich a mixture. It was too much for her immature system to handle. He could have told me that there were other more natural ways to nourish my child. But his only advice was to give her this commercial, processed formula.

In those days, people like me who were exploring a nutrition-oriented, natural approach to health were thought of as fruits and nuts. And we *were* a bit woolly. I mean, after all—dessicated baby veal liver in a baby bottle! But in those days it was either/or. Either you were unquestioningly on the side of traditional medical establishment or you were a ''health food nut.''

Then I found my first nutritionist. I was preparing for *They Shoot Horses, Don't They?,* a movie set in the depression about a dance marathon. People danced at these contests for weeks at a time and the couple who lasted the longest won a lot of prizes, sometimes money. To prepare for our roles, Red Buttons and I decided we would go on the set before the filming began and dance together for a couple of days.

When you have been dancing with someone for hours and hours, you notice a lot of details about him. I think a day had gone by. I was falling asleep, and I could hardly walk. Red Buttons was a good deal older than I but he was not tired. In fact, he was holding me up. My eye was very close to his cheek and I suddenly realized that his skin was unbelievable—rosy and vibrant.

''How come you have such great skin and so much energy?'' I asked. ''What's your secret?''

He told me about his nutritionist in the Valley who advised him on how to eat to improve health and stamina. And that was the doctor who first gave me the helpful sound advice I had been seeking. We should be grateful that it is much easier these days to find a nutritionist.

The way my family and I eat now is diametrically opposed to the wild fluctuations between deprivation and gluttony that marked my early life. I have learned a lot over the years about balance and moderation. I have also learned that you cannot expect your children to be happy eating esoteric beige-colored foods when their friends get soda pop, Snickers and Twinkies.

There was a time when even our birthday cakes were heavy macrobiotic bricks topped with a few strawberries. Nowadays I am more flexible. Our birthdays are sugary celebrations with gooey frosted cakes and ice cream just like everyone else's. Troy and Vanessa have an occasional soft drink and they pig out for days on leftover Halloween candy.

My husband is a real Irish meat-and-potatoes man, but we are trying to cut back on the meat and increase our intake of vegetables and grains. But I don't make any big deal about it. And I don't tell them when I sneak bran or wheat into their scrambled eggs or whip a raw egg into their orange juice.

Instead of being part of the alfalfa sprout fringe-element, I am almost mainstream these days. More people nowadays are interested in good nutrition. It is much easier to find high-quality natural food and herbs than it was ten or fifteen years ago. And it seems to me that more doctors show an interest in the totality of a patient's life, including what they eat and how much they exercise, than they did when Vanessa was a baby.

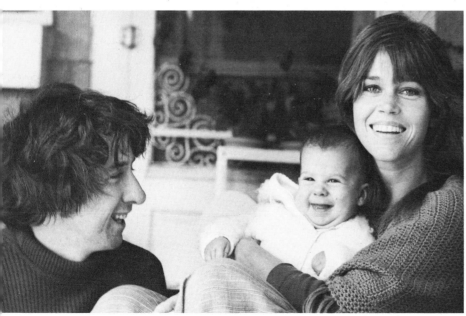

With Tom Hayden and our son, Troy

But there still is a very long way to go. As a nation our consciousnes is not only primitive, it is downright primeval in regard to the effect of nutrition on our total well-being. The majority of us still think of food as a convenience or a panacea. Most of us don't realize how much we can reduce our dependence on doctors and drugs and assume responsibility for our own health if we make nutrition a top priority.

What You Need to Know About Food

Most people know little more about food than they do about their bodies. They know what they like and that's about it. But food is more than a matter of taste—it is the fuel for our bodies. And more than fuel, it maintains and repairs the body. It is only common sense to acquire some basic knowledge about this vital substance. It will take only a short time.

Food provides us with six basic nutrients: proteins, carbohydrates, fats, vitamins, minerals and water. Each has an essential function and each interacts with the others. Enzymes and acids in our digestive system interact with these nutrients, transforming proteins into amino acids, carbohydrates into sugars, and fats into fatty acids and glycerol. In these new forms they are absorbed into the bloodstream.

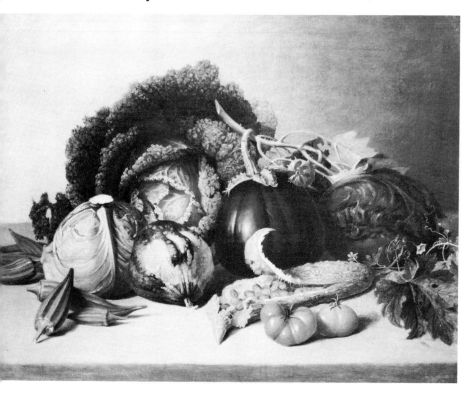

Fats and fat-soluble vitamins go directly from the blood into the cells. The other nutrients go to the liver where still more enzymes alter the chemical composition even further, preparing them to be put to work in cell metabolism. Metabolism is the process by which digested nutrients are converted into building materials for the body's tissue and the production of energy. At all of these stages, enzymes are crucial for proper metabolic function. And all along the way certain vitamins and minerals must be present for the enzymes to do their job.

PROTEIN's primary role is to build, repair and maintain muscle tissue and cells. It also supplies energy when the body's carbohydrate and fat reserves have been exhausted. Such depletion is not desirable, however, since protein cannot be stored and we need it twenty-four hours a day to maintain, rebuild and repair our skin, internal organs, muscles and all the rest. Protein also stimulates hormone production and that of antibodies that fight infections as well as the enzymes that control the chemical reactions in our bodies. If we dip into our protein allowance for energy, these vital processes will suffer.

Proteins are made up of amino acids. There are twenty-three of them altogether, fourteen of which are manufactured by the body. The other nine must be obtained from food. Milk, eggs, meat, fish and poultry give us complete protein with all nine of the essential amino acids that the body does not manufacture. Rice, beans, lentils and wheat germ contain protein, but not all nine essential amino acids. When these foods are properly combined, however—rice with beans, for instance—they make up the nine essential acids.

Most of us were brought up to believe that we need large amounts of protein and that the best way to get it is to eat a lot of meat. Now we are finding out the drawbacks to this kind of diet. We probably eat twice as much protein as our bodies can use. Thirty to fifty grams of protein a day is ample. We will do our bodies the greatest good if we get most of our protein from vegetable rather than animal sources. (The reasons why this is so are discussed in greater detail in the next chapter.) We will also be healthier and stronger if we work out a low-animal-protein, high-natural-carbohydrate diet for ourselves.

CARBOHYDRATES are our chief source of energy. Starch, their main component, is turned into glucose in the body. This glucose provides energy for the brain, the nervous system and the muscles. It is the form of sugar found in the bloodstream and for this reason is often referred to as blood sugar. Some glucose is converted to glycogen and stored within muscle tissue and in the liver. Excess amounts of glucose are stored in the body as fat.

Simple carbohydrates like sugar, corn syrup and honey are turned into glucose rapidly and absorbed directly into the blood. This gives us an immediate energy jolt. But the rapid increase in blood sugar causes the pancreas to quickly produce extra insulin. This triggers a reaction that causes a precipitous drop in blood sugar, leaving us feeling tired—and craving more sweets.

Complex carbohydrates are much better for us. These are found in whole grains, beans, seeds and fresh vegetables. They break down into glucose more slowly, which means that they provide more sustained energy over a greater length of time than simple carbohydrates.

The complex carbohydrates are high in fiber, which is vital for healthy intestines and helps regulate our bowels, reducing the risk of intestinal and rectal cancer. High-fiber foods are digested slowly, which means that their glucose enters the system at a slow rate and gives us a steady, long-term supply of energy.

Highly refined carbohydrates like white flour are low in fiber. Whole wheat bread—the kind that contains the wheat germ and bran—provides eight times more fiber than white bread. I make a habit of adding two tablespoons of unprocessed wheat bran to my food every day and I often sneak some into the scrambled eggs and hamburgers I give my family.

Fiber is also important for people who want to lose weight, because it decreases the amount of calories you absorb from your food. One study, carried out by the Department of Agriculture and the University of Maryland, established that men on a high-fiber diet of 2,500 calories a day absorbed nearly five percent fewer calories than they did on a low-fiber diet of 2,500 calories.

FAT is our second most important source of energy, but a potential dietary time bomb. It supplies nine calories per gram, more than twice as many as proteins and carbohydrates. Whenever we eat more than we need—and it does not matter whether it is carbohydrate or protein or fat—the extra calories are stored in our bodies as fat. Fat also lubricates, insulates, protects our internal organs and provides essential fatty acids.

Generally speaking, we would do well to reduce our intake of all fats, especially saturated animal fats—which are solid at room temperature—including butter, lard, and shortening such as coconut and palm oil. Saturated fat increases the cholesterol level in the blood and the risk of heart disease. It is preferable to use unsaturated fats—which are liquid at room temperature—in the form of vegetable oils like corn oil and safflower oil, in order to minimize the risk of heart disease as well as intestinal and breast cancer. Since vegetable oils become rancid very quickly, it is wise to buy small amounts and keep them in the refrigerator.

VITAMINS—unlike protein, carbohydrates and fat—are not a direct source of energy. They are catalysts for the biochemical reactions that take place in the body. Since some vitamins are not manufactured by the body, we must eat foods that supply them or take vitamin supplements.

If we lived in an unpolluted environment and ate organically grown, unadulterated food, we probably would not need vitamin supplements. But we don't live in a clean environment. Most of us are subject to one form or another of air and water pollution and most of us eat denatured, devitalized food. On top of that, most of the fruits and vegetables sold supermarkets are harvested before they are ripe, transported long di tances and stored before being put on sale. All this results in vitami loss.

Vitamins are either water soluble or fat soluble. The water-soluble v tamins—C and the B family—are not stored in the body, so we mu eat foods that provide them every day. The fat-soluble vitamins—A, [E and K—are stored in the fatty tissues. These can build up to toxi levels in your body if you take too many, but this requires really massiv doses (although A and D vitamin pills are best taken under the guidanc of a doctor).

MINERALS, like vitamins, are needed for many body function especially as building blocks for tissue and as regulators of metaboli processes. We need fourteen different kinds of minerals for good healt and growth, some in large quantities and some, known as trace min erals, in minute amounts.

When you take vitamin and mineral supplements, they should be a least one hundred percent of the recommended daily allowance. Bot vitamin and mineral supplements should be taken with meals. This wa they are absorbed into the system more efficiently.

WATER makes up two-thirds of our body weight. It is required for al most every function from digestion to regulating our temperature t transporting nutrients to removing body wastes.

Most water that is piped into our homes, whether from a municipa water system or from our own wells, contains pollutants such as agri cultural and industrial wastes, chemicals added to destroy bacteria and airborne toxins. I recommend drinking bottled water—natural o distilled. Distilled water lacks minerals, but you can compensate by taking mineral supplements and by eating food rich in minerals such a fresh green vegetables, soybeans, raw, unmilled wheat germ, yeast, al monds, corn, apples, spinach, parsley and watercress.

Fresh fruits and vegetables are excellent sources of pure water, bu we need more than they can supply—a good six to eight glasses daily in addition to whatever fruits and vegetables we eat. It is best to drink water between meals instead of with them so that the digestive juices will not be diluted.

You now have, in the very briefest form possible, a basic under standing of the six main nutrients needed by the body. The quality o the nutrients in the foods that we eat helps determine how well the body's complicated biochemical processes function and whether you will have sustained, high-level energy or have to limp along on the cy clical and debilitating highs and lows of nervous energy.

Eating for Health and Beauty

SEVEN GUIDELINES FOR A HEALTHY DIET

1. Substitute low-fat foods for high-fat foods
2. Cut down on meat—eat low on the food chain
3. Avoid salt and salty foods
4. Cut down on sugar
5. Emphasize whole grains
6. Beware of alcohol
7. Emphasize the Healthy Five:
   Raw unsalted nuts and sesame seeds
   Sprouted seeds such as soybeans
   Fresh raw wheat bran and wheat germ
   Yogurt and kefir
   Fresh fruits and vegetables

As snack foods, processed foods and convenience foods have become the staples of the American diet, they have brought about three significant nutritional changes in our diets.

An increase in the amount of fat we eat. Fat provided 42 percent of the average American's calories in 1976, 31 percent more than in 1910.

A decrease in the amount of complex carbohydrates in our diets. They accounted for only 21 percent of our calories in 1976, 43 percent less than in 1909–1913.

An increase in the amount of sugar we consume. It supplied 18 percent of our calories in 1976, 50 percent more than in 1910.

We can hardly treat ourselves worse. The woman who is concerned about her health and that of her family will substitute high-quality natural foods for low-quality potentially harmful processed and convenience foods. The following seven guidelines for a healthy diet will show you how really simple it can be to eat the high-quality way.

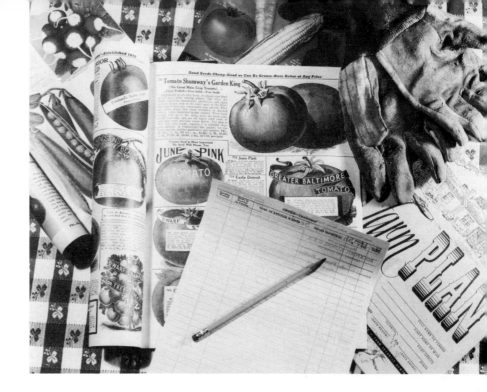

1. SUBSTITUTE LOW-FAT FOODS FOR HIGH-FAT FOODS.

Use skim instead of whole milk. Eat farmer's cheese, cottage cheese, feta and mozzarella instead of high-fat cheeses. In recipes calling for sour cream, use low-fat yogurt. Once you get the substitution habit, you will find dozens of ways to eliminate unhealthy fats from your meals.

2. CUT DOWN ON MEAT.

Frances Moore Lappé, author of *Diet for a Small Planet,* urges us to "eat low on the food chain," because pesticides that do not easily break down accumulate in the fat of animals and fish. When a large fish eats a smaller one, when a cow eats grass or a chicken eats feed, whatever pesticides were present in the smaller fish or grass or feed are retained in the fat of those who are higher up in the food chain. And when we in turn eat fish and meat and poultry, those pesticides start building up in our own bodies. By eating low on the food chain—and that means vegetables and grains—and by sticking to low-fat dairy products, we can reduce the amount of pesticide residues accumulating in our bodies.

The accumulated toxins from the environment are not the only danger in today's meat supply. The way livestock is raised has been fundamentally altered—for the worse. The only one benefiting from the change is the meat supplier.

The deer and the antelope may be the only ones still at home on the range these days. The cattle that once roamed there are now crammed flank to flank into feedlots where they spend their short lives. In the days when they grazed the range, cattle were not considered mature enough to slaughter before they were three or four years old. But in the feedlot where they are under artificial lights twenty-four hours a day nd fed almost constantly, cattle are fattened quickly and cheaply and re slaughtered after eighteen to twenty-five months.

This increased efficiency results in high profits, but it also subjects ie animals to stress and an increased risk of respiratory and other diseases. To minimize these risks and relieve the stress, they are given anti-iotics and tranquilizers. It is estimated that close to 90 percent of the eef and poultry raised for market in this country have been on antibiot-s and other drugs all their lives. Antibiotics as well as synthetic hor-ones and other chemicals are also added to livestock feed to stimu-te growth and weight gain. Their residues are often found in animal ssues—and are not eliminated through cooking.

These "second-hand" doses of antibiotics such as penicillin can pset some people's gastrointestinal processes and cause allergic re-ctions. Health authorities are concerned that constant exposure to ntibiotics in the meat we eat can help disease-causing microbes to uild up immunities, so that if illness strikes these drugs may have lost ieir effectiveness against it.

When livestock is allowed to graze freely and mature naturally the fat tored in their bodies is largely unsaturated. But the fat in feedlot-raised attle is almost entirely saturated. Some health-food stores and butch-rs supply meat from animals that have been raised naturally. If you annot find a source for this meat, at least try to buy fresh meat and in-ist on its being cut in your presence. Ask to see the inspection and rading mark and be sure that all excess fat is trimmed.

The same holds true for poultry. Whenever possible I buy what are alled free-range chickens. Most commercially sold chickens have een raised indoors in such a confined space that they can hardly iove, and have been fed on chemical mush. They have never been out i the sunshine or seen a rooster. Their eggs are infertile.

Free-range chickens are raised outdoors with roosters. They feed on rains, seeds, insects and worms, and are not given synthetic foods or

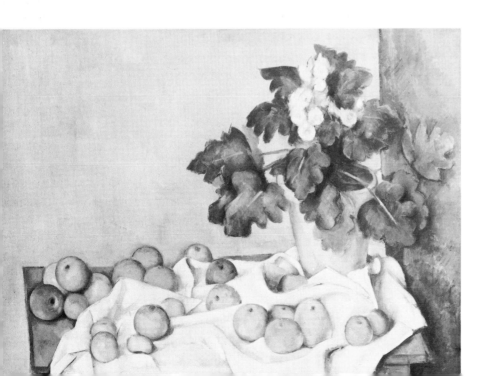

chemicals. Their eggs are fertile and have a higher vitamin content, less saturated fat and a higher nutritional value than those of poultry raised in commercial brooders.

Remember, you do not really need either poultry or meat as long as you eat enough fresh, natural plant protein (beans, brown rice, cereals) and non-meat protein (eggs, milk, cheese). When you do buy meat, choose free-range chickens and turkeys rather than beef. Whenever possible, consider fish as an ideal substitute.

3. AVOID SALT.

This means avoiding salty foods as well. Sodium from salt and additives such as monosodium glutamate increases the risk of developing high blood pressure, which causes some 20,000 deaths a year and is a major factor in 900,000 deaths from stroke and cardiovascular disease every year. Salt also causes fluid retention.

I used to love salt and added it to everything, but during my first pregnancy I went cold turkey and cut it out altogether. It was hard at first, but I soon found I was appreciating the more subtle flavors in food. I have become very sensitive to salt now and do not like the taste any more.

There is enough salt in the foods you eat without having to add more. Don't add it in cooking and don't salt the food on your plate. If you simply *must* salt your food, use Vegit instead, the way we do. This is a powdered herbal and vegetable salt-substitute made by Gayelord Hauser.

4. CUT DOWN ON SUGAR.

Take sugar off your grocery list—and forget about brown sugar too, which does not offer significantly more nutrients than white. If you need a sweetener, use uncooked honey, which besides containing copper, iron, calcium and potassium—in addition to other important minerals—and all nine essential amino acids, is a mild laxative and sedative as well.

Americans now eat 130 pounds of sugar per person a year. This is more than a third of a pound daily for every woman, man and child. Besides being devoid of nutrients, sugar is a full-time promoter of tooth decay, obesity, heart disease and diabetes. It disguises itself cleverly. You will find it listed on labels as corn syrup, dextrose, maltose, glucose and invert sugar.

5. EMPHASIZE WHOLE GRAINS.

If you eat breads and cereals, they should be made of whole grains.

6. BEWARE OF ALCOHOL.

Use it in moderation if at all. It is high in calories, low in nourishment and can cause liver and brain damage.

EMPHASIZE THE HEALTHY FIVE.

The following five groups of foods should be included in your diet as ten as possible:

aw unsalted nuts like almonds, sesame seeds and sunflower seeds. These e high in fiber and packed with vitamins;

orouted seeds such as soybeans, mung beans, alfalfa, which you can sprout ourself at home;

resh, raw wheat bran and wheat germ;

ogurt and kefir, which many people find aid digestion and increase resistance infection;

resh fruits and vegetables and their fresh juices.

If you give yourself just a little time, you will develop a real prefer-nce for natural food. Foods that are adulterated and oversalted will eem revolting. How much more pleasurable a cold, juicy, fresh peach than a soggy, slippery, syrupy canned one! And the canned peach as more calories.

My family and I follow these seven guidelines. Neither our friends nor 1e children's friends seem to notice that there is no white sugar, white read, soda pop or candy in our house except on the most exceptional ccasions like a birthday. Processed foods are at a bare minimum on 1y shelves and sugary breakfast cereals are just not there.

When Tom and I realized that our son, Troy, was singing along with 1e Froot Loops commercial on TV and punctuating every other ad for a ugary cereal with, "Mom, get us some!" we decided to have a little talk rith him. We explained that the big companies that make these prod-cts spend a lot of money trying to persuade children to want these ce-eals so they can make more money. "It's as if they get inside your rain with the commercials," I said, "and make you think these things re good for you even when they're not. So when you watch the com-1ercials, think about what they're trying to put over on you and don't let 1em." He got the message. Not long ago as he was watching a com-1ercial on a children's TV show while I was in the kitchen getting din-er, he called out to me, "They're trying to get inside my mind again, 1om!"

These days Troy is quite satisfied with the Familia, shredded wheat vith added wheat germ, cream of wheat and oatmeal (not the instant ind) that I give him for breakfast.

We eat brown rice instead of the "enriched" white mockery of the tuff and we eat a lot of fresh fruit and drink fresh juices. It is still a bit of battle to get the children to eat a variety of vegetables. Since they oth prefer their vegetables raw, that is how they get them—raw in alads.

After I learned that pasteurization destroys many of the essential vitamins and enzymes in milk, I turned to non-fat certified raw milk instead. Its minerals, protein and fatty acids are easier to digest and assimilate. Thanks to present-day sterilized dairy facilities and refrigeration, one can drink certified raw milk without risk. We have been drinking it for years.

I also use a dietary supplement known as brewer's type yeast flakes. Yeast is a rich source of the B-vitamin complex, magnesium, potassium and calcium. The way I take it is to dissolve several tablespoons of the flakes in a cup of hot water and add a dash of cayenne or capsicum pepper to give it a little zip. It tastes something like chicken broth. I find it is a wonderful energizer, and I drink two or three cups a day instead of coffee.

Unprocessed bran is another important dietary supplement that use. A high-fiber complex carbohydrate, bran is rich in niacin, iron and thiamine.

I always carry my yeast flakes and bran with me when I travel. They seem to help me get over jet lag and make my system feel in balance again. I usually add the bran to yogurt or scrambled eggs.

I like to go to bed slightly hungry and eat a hearty breakfast in the morning. I usually have fresh fruit like melon, strawberries, grapefruit or papaya, and a couple of eggs that I scramble in safflower oil. I may add dried minced onions or fresh herbs and Vegit to them. And I'll have a piece of toast once in a while, made from seven-grain, sprouted wheat or whole wheat bread that contains no preservatives.

Another favorite breakfast of mine is a terrific protein drink. I put some non-fat milk, fresh organic apple juice, strawberries or peaches that I have frozen first, a banana and sometimes a papaya into the blender. I may add wheat germ or bran. And then I add protein powder (When you buy protein powder, try to find one that contains no sugar no preservatives, no artificial colorings or flavor and no soya. The protein powder I use is made from milk and egg protein and I believe it is more easily digested and absorbed by the body than powders made from soya protein.) Then I blend the whole thing until it is smooth and thick. This super fruit milkshake is low in calories, satisfies my sweet tooth and usually fills me up so I don't want to eat again until the middle of the afternoon.

This raises the question of when you should eat. My recommendation is that you should eat only when you are hungry—not because it is one o'clock or seven o'clock or whatever. There is research which indicates that what you eat early in the day is less fattening than what you eat at night. The reason is that your body functions differently at night. If you have your major meal during the day, it will be absorbed while your blood circulation is active. But if you eat a large meal in the evening, the fatty contents of your meal will be absorbed by a sluggish bloodstream. It also forces your digestive system to work overtime while you sleep.

There is another good reason for having your major meal during the day. If you have eaten lightly all day, your blood sugar will be low at night and you will probably eat more than you need. In other words, you will binge. And if you are trying to lose weight, you have defeated yourself. All that depriving yourself during the day is canceled by overeating at night.

One of the great dieting booby traps is the need you may feel for a pick-me-up during the day. It usually comes around the same time, which means that your blood sugar level has dropped. This happens to everyone at some time, but it is accentuated when you diet. Your impulse is to reach for something sugary for quick energy. And that is the worst thing you can do to yourself.

I protect myself against the sugar urge by carrying an apple or some other fresh fruit with me. The natural sugar in the fruit will raise my blood sugar level, appease my hunger the natural way and give me energy without the high jolt of refined sugar and the precipitous, almost sickening drop that follows.

The woman who wants to eat for health and also wants to lose weight should understand that there is really only one way to do it. You must decrease the amount of food you eat and increase the amount of exercise you get. That is all there is to it. Starving, crash diets or subsisting on small amounts of junk food is not the way to lose weight. You will gain the pounds back as soon as you return to your normal eating habits. When food becomes the enemy with which we are locked in an obsessive power struggle, then every time we lose the fight we not only gain weight but we lose our self-esteem as well. I know. I've been there.

The best and easiest way to change your attitude about food is to put it in its proper place. Think of it as it really is—fuel for your body. So instead of focusing your anxieties on food call off the fight, declare a truce and accept food as a life-giving friend. When you are dieting you want to give your body the best fuel available—which means food that is low in calories, but natural and wholesome and as free from contaminants as possible. Your best course is to eat the high-fiber, complex-carbohydrate, low-animal-protein, low-fat diet that I have described in this chapter. Just eat less of it and increase your exercise.

Whether or not you are on a diet, I suggest that the woman who wants to eat for health and beauty make a habit of reading food labels before she buys any processed food. This is the easiest way to know what you will actually be eating. Once you read the label, you might just change your mind and put the processed food right back on the shelf.

Labels give the ingredients in descending order of the amounts, so if sugar is the first or second ingredient listed, you just know that that food, whatever it is, does not belong on a health diet. You should also avoid products that contain such questionable additives as nitrates, saccharin, sodium, artificial colorings and petroleum additives such as BHA and BHT.

There has been conclusive evidence in the last few years that a few of the chemical additives in our food, acting alone or when combined with other chemicals in the stomach, can cause cancer. Some of the chemicals that appear to promote cancer include saccharin, sodium nitrite, BHT and red dye No. 40.

In response to the studies showing these additives to be carcinogens, the food industry argues that the doses administered to the rats in the tests were much larger than humans would ever ingest, their assumption being that a small dose of a cancer-causing substance poses no risk. But cancer experts maintain there are no safe doses of carcinogens. If a large amount of a substance can cause cancer, then a small amount of the same substance can also cause cancer—but less often or over a longer span of time.

The experts believe there may be a threshold for carcinogen exposure, that small doses of a substance accumulate over time and that even a very weak dose of a carcinogen may be all that is needed to push the body's total carcinogenic burden over the threshold into cancer.

We are all exposed to carcinogens every day. From some foods (moldy peanuts, for instance); from air and water pollution; from X rays and the ultra-violet rays of the sun. These exposures alone could bring your body near its carcinogen threshold. We can do nothing about some of these exposures, but why should we increase our risk of cancer by knowingly ingesting even a small amount of a proven carcinogen? It could be the straw that breaks the camel's back.

I urge you to respect the complexities of your biochemical processes, which directly affect your moods, your health and your energy-level. The woman who respects the needs of her body will junk the junk food and start eating foods that are as close to their natural living or growing state as possible.

She will teach her children to respect their bodies and eat only the foods that are good for them. Tom and I have spent a lot of time explaining to Vanessa and Troy why we ask them to eat more of some things and less of others. We have explained why the red coloring in the maraschino cherries they love is dangerous for them and that the sodium nitrite which is used to preserve, color and flavor hot dogs can cause cancer. We have found that when they really understand what is good and bad for them, they tend to guide themselves.

I remember, for instance, going to a movie with them. We hadn't had lunch yet and were hungry so I asked if they wanted a hot dog. Vanessa put her hands on her hips and said, ''Mm-o-om,'' turning it into a three-syllable word the way she does when she disapproves of me. ''You know they're bad for us.''

''Hallelujah!'' I thought.

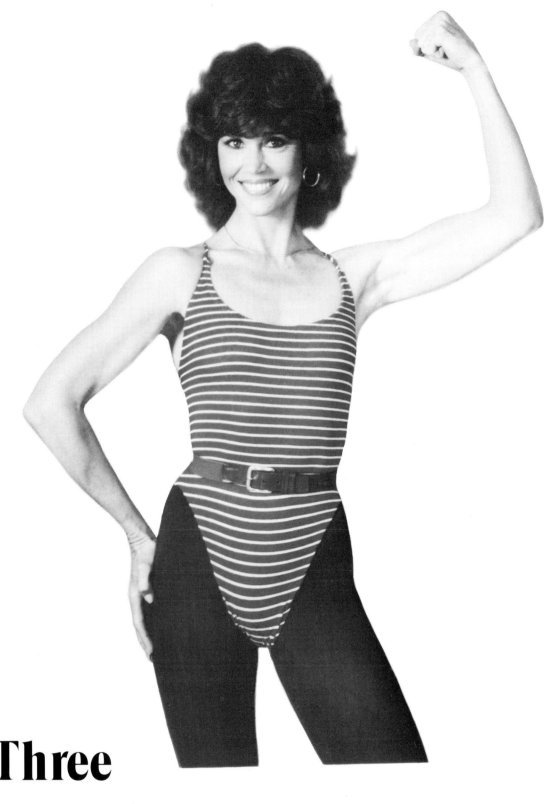

Part Three
Being Strong

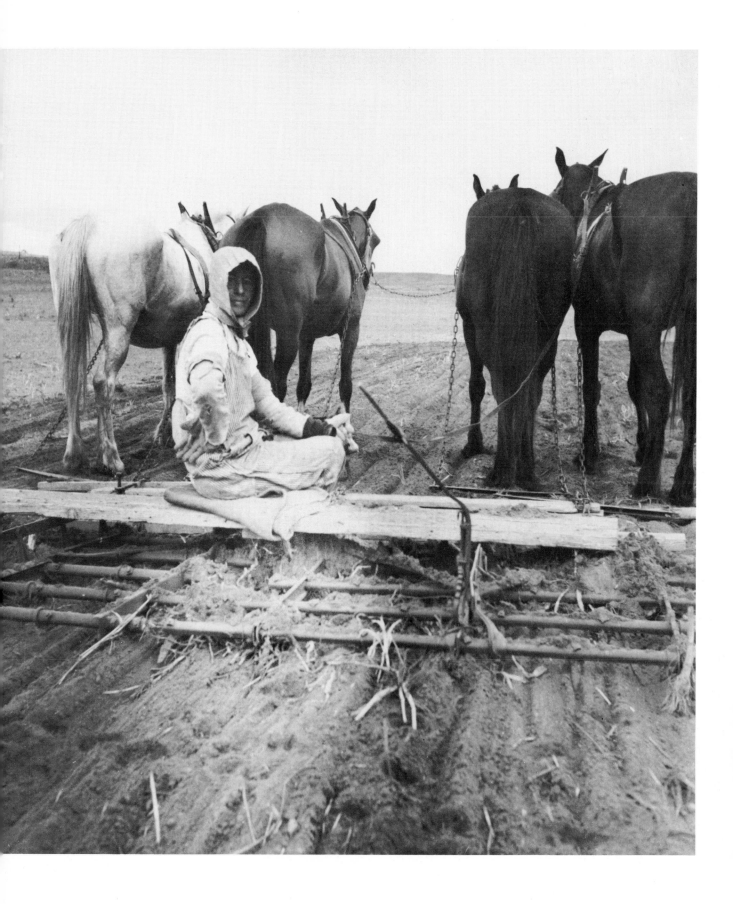

Breaking the
"Weaker Sex" Mold

There was a time when heavy physical work was an accepted part of both men's and women's lives. Women had to be strong because they bore an equal share of the burden of providing for the family.

Many of us in this country are descendants of pioneer women who worked shoulder-to-shoulder with their men to push back the wilderness, build homesteads, plow the virgin prairies. One of my ancestors, Peggy Fonda, lived in Fonda, a hamlet in upstate New York, to which the Dutch Fondas had emigrated in 1642. In order to provide General Washington's army with flour, this lady—a widow—rebuilt the family gristmill with her own two hands after it was burned to the ground during the Revolution. There were thousands and thousands of women like her, grittily strong and courageous.

In the days before the Industrial Revolution of the nineteenth century, only the women of the aristocracy were required to be fragile, ornamental testaments to their husband's wealth and power. The Industrial Revolution transformed the lives of the laboring class, taking them out of the fields and moving them into the factories that were spawned by the new machine technology. The men of the emerging middle class flaunted their new status by employing servants to do the work wives had done before. And a century later, they bought gadgets and appliances to replace the servants.

Strong backs and muscles were no longer valued in women. The cultural ideal of a desirable woman was one who was delicate and decorative, like her aristocratic sisters. And this is the ideal that we have all internalized to some extent.

During World War II, when women had to fill the jobs of the men who had gone to war as well as provide the working force for the new booming war industries, this concept of fragile femininity was conveniently

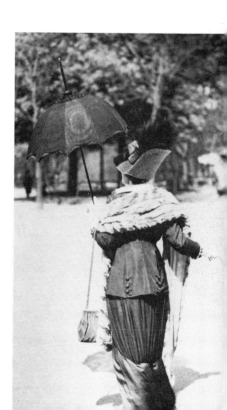

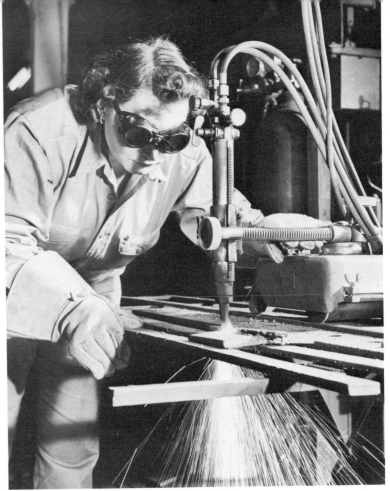

Woman welder during World War II

altered almost overnight. Rosie the Riveter became a heroine. I have an image in my mind from the forties of powerful-looking women with broad shoulders, heads wrapped in scarves, working on an assembly line.

Breast-feeding suddenly became unfashionable, discouraged because it kept women pinned down at home. Day-care centers were funded so that women who would otherwise have stayed home taking care of their children could join the labor force. The strong independent woman was suddenly trotted out again as a role model, lauded in movies, novels, songs and advertisements, because the country needed her.

No sooner was the war over, however, and the men streaming back to civilian life and their old jobs, than women were once again relegated to the category of "the weaker sex." The same media voices that had saluted the independent woman now deplored the situation of the "eight-hour orphans" who were being "neglected" by their working mothers.

Today women are becoming strong again. We are rejecting the equation of femininity with weakness at every level, including the physical. Once again, economic factors are involved. Inflation has forced wives to assume a share of their husband's financial burden in order to meet the basic needs of their families. Half the married women in this country now work outside the home. There is also a large population of divorced, widowed and single women who must support themselves and often their children. The economics of health care are such that these women cannot afford to be sick. They *have* to keep themselves strong and healthy.

There is also the problem of just plain physical safety. Women are often frightened to go out at night, not only in the large cities, but in our small towns and suburbs as well. I am not exaggerating. According to a very conservative estimate, a woman is raped every other minute. And rape represents only one category of physical attack upon women. The YWCA recently completed a nationwide survey which revealed that 20 million women a year are physically abused by their husbands or lovers. Concern for our physical safety is forcing us to work at making our bodies capable of responding quickly in emergencies, defending ourselves, or running fast enough to get away if we are attacked.

But I do not see the emergence of today's strong and healthy women simply as a repeat of the previous patterns of economic determinism that have dictated the role of women over the centuries, nor as a pragmatic and visceral response to fear. This time women are taking the initiative, they are not being manipulated.

The new female consciousness that has developed over the last decade extends to our right to physical as well as economic, political and social equality. We not only need to develop and extend our physical limits, we want to. And we refuse to be afraid that we will no longer be considered attractive and acceptable when we are strong. We now recognize the strong, healthy woman who has fulfilled her physical potential, as beautiful. And she is. Gayle Olinekova, marathon runner; Mary Decker, world champion runner; Nadia Comaneci, Olympic gymnast; Beth Heiden, champion skater and cyclist; Evelyn Ashford, runner; and

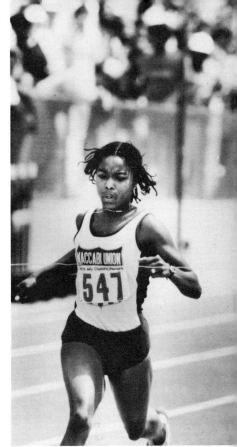

Evelyn Ashford

Gayle Olinekova

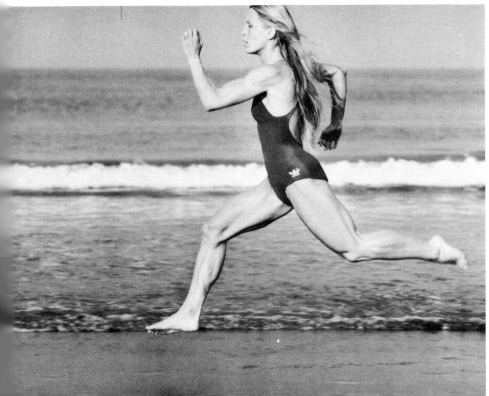

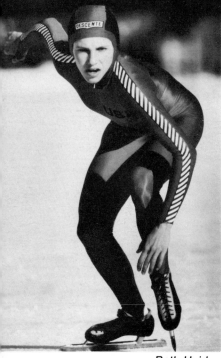

Beth Heiden

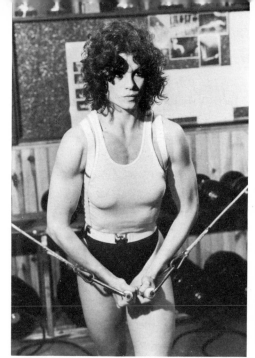

Lisa Lyon

Mary Decker

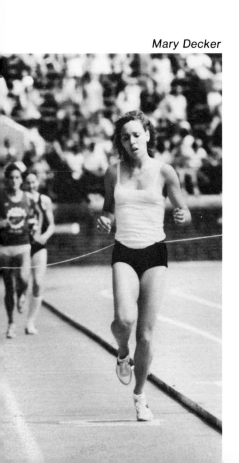

Lisa Lyon, world champion bodybuilder, are just a few examples of women who are strong and beautiful.

And then there is Janice Darling. She is an actress and has worked as an instructor at the Workout Studio. If you turn to pages 98 through 102, you'll see Janice demonstrating exercises. She has taught all of us who know her what it means to be strong in the full sense of the word.

Less than six months before those pictures were taken, Janice was standing in line outside a movie theater when a speeding car went out of control and drove up onto the sidewalk. Janice was hurled through a plate-glass storefront. Her pelvis was crushed, both her legs were broken and a piece of glass flew into her left eye and severed the eye muscle.

Janice spent a month in the hospital. The doctors told her it would be many more months before she could walk. She refused to accept this and set about an intensive program of self-rehabilitation. She had friends bring her yogurt and high-protein energy drinks (if you stay in a hospital more than two weeks, you run a very real risk of malnutrition). And she asked for a taped exercise program. Even though she was confined to her hospital bed, she managed to devise a special exercise regime for her upper body and torso. To strengthen her legs, she did the exercises with weights strapped to her ankles.

The doctors and nurses were amazed at her determination—and at how quickly she recovered. She was back teaching at the Workout Studio in four months. She has a prosthetic eye and wears an eye patch that she says ought to give her a crack at more exotic roles. "Being in good shape is not just looking good," Janice says. "A good physical condition is protection. Our strength comes from our body. The fact that I was hit by a car and not torn to pieces or killed is proof of that. My muscles were so toned and so strong they literally saved my life!"

Most of us want to be strong, but we are not. Automation, automobiles, sedentary jobs and sexual stereotyping have all had a destructive impact on our bodies. Did you know that the typical job in a modern office (where most women work) requires less physical exertion than taking a shower? I don't mean to suggest there is anything wrong with automation and labor-saving devices. I, for one, would not want to return to the scrubbing board and butter churn. But while enjoying these conveniences we ought to take advantage of the increased leisure time they give us to engage in some form of physical activity. Our bodies were meant to be used and used hard. Our muscle structure needs to be strengthened and toned so that it can support our skeletal structure properly and protect our spines.

Without proper exercise, we are likely to age prematurely and suffer from hypertension, loss of flexibility and muscle tone, lower back problems, heart problems, excess weight, chronic fatigue and depression. (Incidentally, depression is a major cause of overeating.) Doctors recommend exercise for varicose veins, arthritis, migraine, menstrual cramps and nicotine craving. It has been shown that exercise decreases the level of cholesterol in your blood.

The feelings of elation and bursting energy that you get when you exercise hard are not mystical. Vigorous exercise produces chemicals in the body that act as natural anti-depressants. Psychiatrists know that exercise has a therapeutic effect on people suffering from mental disorders. I have found that I think more clearly when I've worked out because my blood is carrying more oxygen to my brain. Notice I've said "vigorous" and "exercise hard." I don't use these words idly. Namby-pamby little routines that don't speed up your heart beat and make you sweat aren't really worth your while. For it to matter—from both a health and esthetic point of view—you have to make an effort, put your heart into it. Literally!

Exercise won't remove freckles or make your feet smaller or your eyes bigger. But, rosy-cheeked and clear-eyed, you will laugh more, step livelier, and speak out with assertiveness. You will like yourself more and you will enjoy loving more. The color of the leaves will please you more. So will the feel of crisp cool air on your skin. You'll be more attentive to little changes in nature that you used to pass right by. Best of all, you may rediscover the child in you who was lost along the way.

I do not claim that a strong, healthy woman is automatically going to be a progressive, decent sort of person. Obviously other factors are involved in that. But I am sure that one's innate intelligence and instinct for good can be enhanced through fitness.

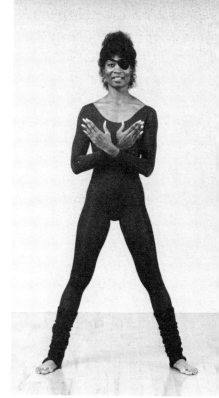

Janice Darling

Nadia Comaneci

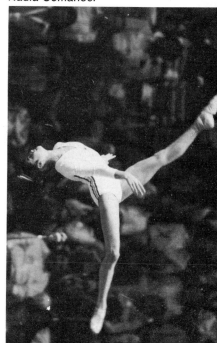

The Natural Approach to Weight Loss

One out of every three Americans is overweight. Aside from the emotional and psychological problems this may present, excess weight is a real health hazard. For one thing, your heart has to work harder to pump blood through all that fatty tissue, and this can lead to high blood pressure.

Too little exercise is as much to blame for excess weight as too much food. You can lose weight by dieting, but much of the weight loss on a short diet is really water loss. This is quickly replaced when you resume normal eating and drinking. Strict and prolonged diets expose you to nutritional problems. Then, too, a full quarter of your weight loss on such extreme diets will be due to loss of muscle tissue. If you then go off your diet, and start eating more calories than you use up, the weight you gain will be fat, with the result that you will have more fat and less muscle than before you started dieting. You will tend to be more tired and less active—and will gain even more weight.

The fastest, healthiest, and most effective, interesting and rewarding way to lose weight is by combining vigorous exercise with a healthful diet. The key is to find the balance between the calories you take in and the ones you burn up. The best results come when you simultaneously cut down on caloric intake and increase the calories you burn up through exercise.

"But exercise makes me so hungry! I'll gain weight, not lose it," many women have told me. This is not true. Carefully controlled medical studies have shown that for the average person, the *opposite* is true. A lean, trim woman who exercises vigorously will burn up stored fat and will tend to eat more after her workout to replace the calories she has burned up, but most people have large stores of fat and the amount of exercise they do does not stimulate the appetite.

My own experience, which has been proven empirically over and over again by clients at my Workout Studios, is that exercise depresses

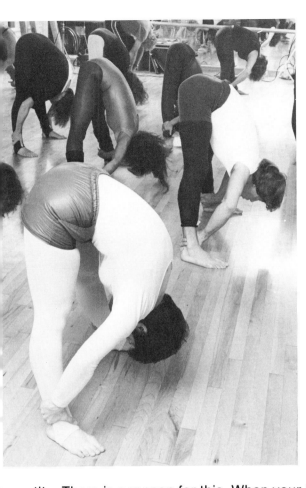

appetite. There is a reason for this. When your blood-sugar level drops, you feel hungry. If you exercise regularly, your blood-sugar level will remain stable because your muscles will be using proportionately more fat than sugar as fuel. And there is less insulin in your blood. As I explained earlier, insulin causes the blood-sugar level to drop rapidly and this makes you feel hungry. So you do not need to be afraid that exercising will stimulate your appetite and result in your gaining weight. Quite the opposite. Exercise also makes food pass through the digestive tract more rapidly so that fewer calories are absorbed from what you do eat.

Exercise affects your metabolism, the combustion process that takes place within the cells when carbohydrates in the form of glucose or glycogen and oxygen are burned to create energy. The energy that is released during this process is measured in calories. This is what is meant by ''burning up calories.''

Your metabolic rate increases during vigorous exercise and it takes considerable time to slow down again afterwards. This means that you will continue to burn calories even after you stop exercising. And the greater the ratio of lean tissue to body fat, the more calories you will burn, because lean tissue is more highly oxygenated than fat and thus keeps the metabolic process going longer.

If you exercise long enough at one time, your muscles will begin to use fat for fuel instead of carbohydrates, almost as if they said, "Hey, the carbohydrates are getting low. I guess we better start burning up some of that stored fat instead." In the process, your muscles are being programmed to store carbohydrates while burning fat, thereby increasing your endurance.

Steve Kelly, three-time member of the U.S. Olympic kayak team and manager of the Sports Training Institute in Manhattan, where serious athletes as well as people interested in keeping fit work out, says that the stored fat does not start to be burned until you have exercised vigorously for at least an hour. But when you do start to burn it, that fat comes from deposits all through your body. The fat is mobilized into the bloodstream and carried to the muscle cells that need fuel for energy. This is the reason why the experts insist that there is no such thing as spot reducing. Maybe. But something certainly happens to those saddle bags, dingle-dangles, love handles and plain old lumps and bumps. Basically it is a matter of muscle toning and tightening, which shrinks the size of the fatty deposits that some people call cellulite. Fat accumulates in areas where the muscles are unused and the metabolism sluggish. When you start working these muscles, the metabolism wakes up. The muscle cells need energy, so more blood is pumped there with more oxygen for the metabolic process and for carrying away the toxins that accumulate.

You may have been exercising vigorously and watching your diet but the pounds are just not coming off. Be patient. Each body responds differently to exercise. It depends on what you eat, how out of shape you were before you started and how hard you work at your exercising. Some people may be rewarded with instant weight loss—and then stay at the same weight for weeks.

There are reasons why weight loss may be slow. As you begin to burn up fat for muscle fuel, your body tends to retain water. This water weight will come off through the elimination of the excess fluid as sweat and urine. You also have to take into account the fact that muscle weighs more than fat and takes up less space. You will probably find that you lose inches before you start losing pounds. The secret of losing weight is patience, regular vigorous exercise and the determination to push yourself beyond what you were able to do yesterday.

As we grow older, the amount of fat in our bodies tends to increase because our metabolism slows down. And we usually are less active physically. If we keep eating the same amount of food that we did when we were younger, we will gain weight. It is particularly important, therefore, for women over thirty to find the balance between intake and output.

You need to eat only a few extra calories a day to be very sorry in a few years. If you eat 100 calories more than you burn up every day, you can expect to have gained more than 50 pounds at the end of five years. But if you had exercised just a little more every day—taken a risk half-hour walk or bicycled for twenty minutes or jogged for an extra ten minutes or so—those 50 extra pounds would not have accumulated. Knowing this, and really understanding it, should liberate you from an obsession with dieting—which really means an obsession with eating—from fear of gaining weight, and from the sense of defeat you have when you fail to stick to a diet. Strenuous exercisers, myself included, can eat more and carry more weight without showing it than we could in our pre-workout days. We can eat normally, even indulge in chocolate cake or pecan pie or whatever once in a while as long as we are prepared to work out a little longer, sweat a little more the next day.

Exercise teaches you the pleasure of discipline and, if you can discipline yourself to an exercise program, it's easier to exert discipline over your eating habits. You feel more in control of your compulsions instead of being controlled by them. Instead of taking the purely negative approach of self-denial—"I *won't* eat this, I *won't* eat that"—you're doing something *positive* for yourself and, believe me, the more you treat yourself positively, the less you'll want or need to be negative.

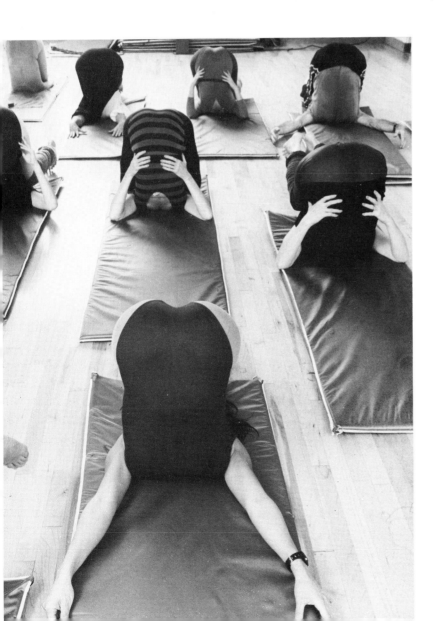

Making a Commitment

A commitment to exercise regularly and vigorously is not easy. I would never try to pretend otherwise. When I think about this business of commitment and discipline, I think of Katharine Hepburn and the summer of 1980.

We were filming *On Golden Pond* in New Hampshire. At one point I was supposed to do a back flip into the freezing cold water of Squam Lake. I had never even done a back dive before, much less a back flip. And as a Californian who hates cold water, I was not at all sure that this Fonda dog was not too old to learn new tricks. It would have been perfectly reasonable to have a stunt woman do the back flip for me. Why not?

Then I met Miss Hepburn. She asked if I intended to learn how to do a back flip, and she let it be known that *she* could do one. I found out

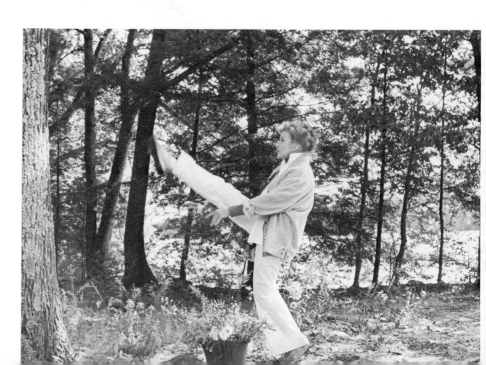

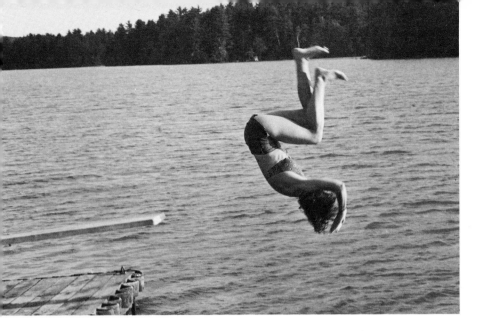

hat she had been a competitive diver at one time, and then I remembered that great dive she made in *Philadelphia Story*. I felt challenged, and I must confess that I wanted her to like me, so I decided that I would try to learn to do a back flip.

Day after day that summer I practiced with a wonderful instructor. First in a pool and then from a float in Squam Lake. I was lousy. My legs would slam against the water so hard they stung and were bruised. All my adolescent convictions about being a klutz came back in waves. It got so that I was terrified every time I tried that flip, but I did not want to lose Miss Hepburn's respect, so I kept going.

I finally mastered it. Nothing to write home about, but it was a back flip, and I could do it. One day as I was climbing out of that icy water, Miss Hepburn approached me. "Don't you feel good?" she asked with that smile.

"Just terrific," I said. And I did. Miss Hepburn must have recognized the way I felt, because she said, "Everyone should know that feeling of overcoming fear and mastering something. People who aren't taught that become soggy!"

Katharine Hepburn is the least soggy person I know. That summer at Squam Lake she told me of the pleasure she has in extending herself physically. In her seventies she is a testament to non-sogginess. I certainly will be less soggy as a result of knowing her. She made me realize that it is never too late to master your weaknesses and feel the elation that comes with pushing yourself to new levels. You may be soggy today, but there is no reason for you to be soggy tomorrow.

If you are serious about wanting to lose weight once and for all, about changing the shape of your body, about improving your self-image and your morale, you must get over being soggy. There are no short cuts. No sweatless quickies. You must be committed to working hard, sweating hard and getting sore. You cannot do it passively by going to a spa and having your bottom jiggled on a vibrating belt, taking a few swipes at bicycling and sitting in a sauna. All you are doing is fooling yourself and wasting your money.

You have to work for it. The ideal is to do some form of vigorous exercise every day. If you cannot find time to exercise every day, then you have to make up in intensity and duration what you lose in frequency. The absolute minimum for effective exercise is three times a week or alternate days for at least half an hour a day. As you continue, your body will start to tell you when you can do more. I don't feel that I have pushed myself hard enough if I work out for less than an hour, but I am accustomed to exercise. Forty minutes may be your limit, or even thirty. Don't place unreasonable demands on yourself. It is important to try to do more and better each time, but let your body be your guide.

If you expect more of yourself than you are capable of doing, it can be counterproductive. The guilt you feel when you can't live up to your unreasonable demands may send you right back to a soggy way of life. Build up your strength gradually. Don't push yourself so hard at the beginning that you are panting and gasping.

There is no reason why vigorous exercise cannot be a regular part of your life. I have a frantically busy schedule, with long erratic hours of work, plus children, a husband, a house to run—the works. But for the past fifteen years, I have made fitness a priority, because I have experienced its very real rewards. I simply schedule it into my life as if my life depended on it, which in a way it does. I do it for myself and I do it no matter what.

It is not easy. You will always have a good reason to skip your workout. You could be cleaning the house, baking, watching a movie, going straight home from work or sleeping late. But when you make yourself exercise and afterwards feel that tingle through your body, the sense of exhilaration and your own pleasure in your discipline, you'll agree it was worth it. Whatever it was that you did not do in order to make time to work out, you can do now—and probably do it better.

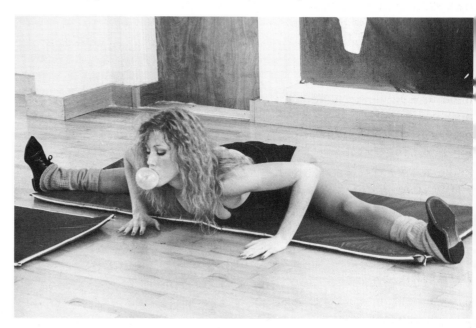

Choosing What You Do

The kind of exercise you choose will depend in part on the facilities available to you, whether there is a track, jogging route, swimming pool, gym or stimulating dance or exercise class in your neighborhood.

You also have to consider any physical problems you have. If you have a serious back problem, I suggest you consult a chiropractor about what exercises you can and cannot do. If you are significantly overweight, or have any indication of heart problems, you should have your blood pressure checked and an electrocardiogram taken. You can still exercise, in fact exercise will be beneficial, but you should be prudent and exercise only under strict and informed supervision.

The exercise program you set up for yourself should include aerobics for cardiovascular conditioning and endurance, resistance exercises to increase your muscle strength and stretching for flexibility. My own Workout program, which I outline in detail in Part IV, fits my needs in all three areas, but everyone has her own temperament and body rhythm, so when you develop your own exercise program, listen to your body.

If you are going to stick with your workout program—and I think of mine as a lifetime commitment—it has to be something that suits you and that you enjoy. Enjoyable does not necessarily mean easy. The joy comes from accomplishing something you did not think you could do before—like that back flip I mastered, for instance. It comes from knowing that you are not, in Katharine Hepburn's word, soggy.

But whatever type of workout you settle on, it should include the Big Three of exercise for health and fitness—aerobics, resistance exercises and stretching.

AEROBICS

Walking briskly, jogging, running, cross-country skiing, swimming, cycling, jumping rope and vigorous, non-stop exercises are aerobic activi-

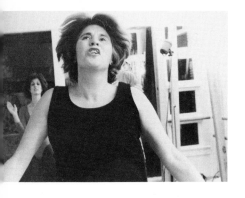

ties. They are rhythmic, sustained and use the large muscle groups, particularly those in the hips and legs. This is why aerobic exercise promotes cardiovascular fitness and endurance.

The way it works is that the rhythmic contractions of the large hip and leg muscles press against the blood vessels so that they send increased amounts of blood to the heart. This makes the heart work harder. The heart is a muscle and, like any muscle, becomes larger and stronger when it is made to work harder—but only to a certain percentage of its capacity and for a carefully controlled length of time.

As the heart muscle becomes stronger, it pumps more oxygen-carrying blood through the vascular system with fewer beats. When more blood is pumped through your system, more oxygen is available for the production of energy.

As with any combustion engine, the process of burning fuel to provide energy requires oxygen. Aerobic exercise causes the arteries to enlarge, increases the number of capillaries (the smallest blood vessels) that bring blood to the muscles, increases the number of oxygen-carrying cells in your blood and improves the ability of the enzymes in your muscles to extract the oxygen from your blood.

To achieve true aerobic fitness, you must increase your heart rate to a training level and sustain that training level for a minimum of twenty minutes at least three times a week.

You can determine your own training level by first figuring out your maximum heart rate. The maximum rate at which a heart can beat is 220 beats a minute, but that rate decreases by one beat for every year of life. To get your own maximum heart rate, subtract your age from 220. If you are thirty, it will be 190 (220 – 30 = 190). If you are forty, it will be 180.

Your training level is between 70 and 85 percent of your maximum heart rate. If you are thirty, your training level will be between 133 and 162 beats a minute. If you are forty, it will be between 126 and 153.

To find out if you are exercising at your training level, you should take your pulse after you have been exercising hard for several minutes. Take your pulse for six seconds and then multiply the count by 10

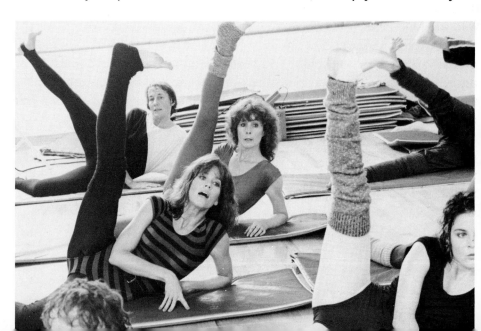

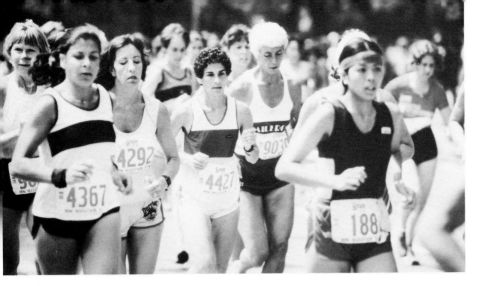

to get your heartbeat per minute. If you have not exercised for a long time and/or are out of shape, you should begin at the 60 percent level and work up to the 70 and then to the 85 percent levels very, very gradually.

Running is an excellent form of aerobic exercise that costs nothing and can be done almost anywhere——on the high-school track, on a quiet suburban street, along a country road, on the beach, in the park, even around your house or driveway or the supermarket parking lot before the supermarket opens in the morning.

There was a time when I never dreamed I could jog or run. I had gone running a few times with men, but every time my chest would ache and I would be gasping for breath within minutes. I had also heard that running gave you big leg muscles, made your bottom drop and was bad for a woman's reproductive organs. That settled it. Running was not for me.

Then about two years ago, I tried again. Three women friends who were regular runners invited me to go running with them one evening. They were going to run along the Pacific Palisades, a beautiful stretch that overlooks the ocean near where we live. I was surprised at how easy it was. We ran along chatting with each other and when we started to pant, we would stop and walk. I suddenly realized that I loved it. I felt great. And so proud of myself! I could do it! I realized that I had been doing it wrong before because I was trying to run too fast, competing with men who were experienced runners.

After this experience, I took running seriously. I started very slowly and when I began to pant, I dropped down to a brisk walk for a while and then jogged again. Little by little my jogging time grew longer and the walking time shorter. I was really excited when I jogged my first mile.

When I finally reached the two-mile mark, I got too cocky. The next day I abruptly increased my distance to three miles and began running three miles a day every day at a time when I was very tired. I paid for this mistake with a painful "runner's knee" and could not run for three weeks.

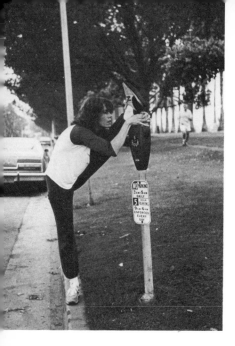 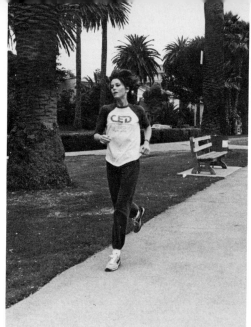 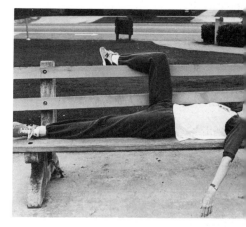

This started me reading books on running, something I encourage you to do before you start running yourself. I learned that it was important to increase distance gradually, that one should not be compulsive about running the maximum distance every day and that it was important to listen to one's body. If it tells you that you are tired, don't push too hard.

About this time I came upon a poem by Lao Tzu whose wisdom I now try to keep in mind.

For all things there is a time for going ahead and a time for following behind,
A time for slow breathing and a time for fast breathing,
A time to grow in strength and a time to decay,
A time to be up and a time to be down.
Therefore, the sage avoids all extremes, excesses and extravagances.

As for all those dire forecasts that I used to believe about running—well, it may not be the ideal exercise for some people, because it does put stress on your knee and hip joints. And it may not be indicated for women with fragile reproductive organs. I am not qualified to say. I do know, however, that if you have the proper running shoes and come down on your heels first rather than your toes, you will not build large leg muscles nor will your bottom drop. On the contrary, the muscles in your buttocks, hips, thighs and legs are being strengthened, and, judging from my own experience, if you keep your pulse rate up to your training level long enough, you will be shedding fat in those problem areas. Your muscles will stay long and flexible and you'll have less risk of injury if you take a few minutes to warm up and stretch before and after your run.

I love running now. I try to do six or seven miles several times a week and three or four miles on off-days. I have run through the dappled summer light of country roads in New England, chugged around indoor tracks so small that I felt like a hamster on an exercise wheel, run in Central Park in New York when it was so cold my tears froze, and dragged myself bleary-eyed into the California dawn to get my run in before the children woke up.

I love that it gets me outside and turns my skin pink all over. I enjoy seeing the familiar faces of fellow runners, particularly those feisty over-60s. I like that it is free, that you can do it anywhere, and I especially love it when it's over.

MACHINES: PASSIVE RESISTANCE

It seems most of my new exercise experiences happen as a result of breaking my feet. One broken foot got me started with my Workout regime. Another time when I was in Israel I broke my foot late at night running to answer the telephone in a strange apartment. I turned the wrong way and fell downstairs. This happened only weeks before I had to begin filming *On Golden Pond,* where once more I had to wear a bikini—and do that back flip. I could not afford to wait until the cast came off to get into shape. There just wasn't time. I had to start practically immediately, cast be damned!

I went to classes at my Workout Studio and did what I could with that big plaster lump weighing me down. But it wasn't enough. In desperation I went to a gym which was equipped with Nautilus machines.

The whole notion of using machines and weights left me cold. They seemed absolutely contrary to my dancer's sensibilities. I soon learned, however, that many dancers use machines, and they are uniquely helpful for anyone with an injury. Each machine uses isolated muscle groups so you can quite safely work your body while avoiding the injured area.

There are different kinds of equipment—Nautilus, Universal, Camm II and others. You can get a good workout on all of them if you know how to use them. It really depends on which equipment is most convenient for you. Nautilus has been the most accessible for me.

Each Nautilus machine works a specific muscle group. You perform an exercise or a movement that forces the muscle to use its full range of motion against resistance provided by the machine. You do each movement until you reach the point of momentary muscular failure when the build-up of lactic acid prevents further muscle contraction.* Then you go on to another exercise that works another muscle group.

I am disturbed by how often I see people using the machines incorrectly because they are not getting the most out of the time and energy they are spending. Ideally, you should have a trainer with you when you use the machines, but this is expensive. In New York, when I was making *Rollover* in the spring of 1981 and using the machines at the Sports Training Institute, it cost ten dollars a session for a trainer. But I think it is worth it, at least in the beginning while you are learning to use the machines. If the gym you go to does not provide individual training, try to find a trainer somewhere else who can spend time giving you thorough instruction before you go it alone.

When I began with the Nautilus, I worked to build my strength and used the maximum amount of weight I could manage. When I got

* For an explanation of the cause and significance of this momentary muscle failure (it is nothing to worry about), see page 68.

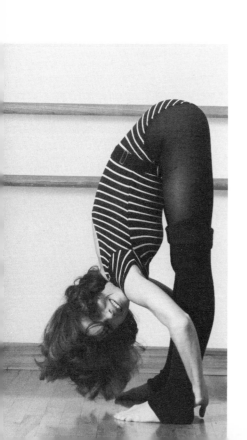

stronger my trainer at the Sports Training Institute, marathon cyclist David White, changed my program so that I was working more for endurance. Now he has me do several sprints on a stationary bicycle to get my pulse rate up to training level. Then I begin the exercises on the machines, moving from one exercise to the next with little or no rest in between so that my pulse rate never has a chance to drop below my training level. My trainer will have me do sit-ups and push-ups between some of the exercises to keep my pulse rate up. The overall routine is very fast, but the exercises themselves are never rushed. I try to perform them smoothly and steadily. I like this aerobic type of Nautilus workout because it provides cardiovascular conditioning while increasing my strength.

A beginner should be warned against attempting the kind of workout that I have just described. You must build up to it gradually. Besides that, working out on machines is such a high-intensity effort that you should do it only every other day. Otherwise, you become susceptible to injury. The muscle fibers, which have been worked to the point of failure, need time to repair themselves and replenish their fuel supply.

When I first started training on the Nautilus equipment (and after my foot had healed), I became too gung ho. I went to the gym two days in a row, did my regular workout and ran each day. I was not just sore as a result, I was so tired it was hard to get out of bed, and so depressed that I did not want to anyway. I discovered these are classic symptoms of overtraining.

Incidentally, if you have gone off your exercise routine for a week or more, don't try to jump right back in at the same level. Your muscles will have lost some of their ability to use oxygen efficiently. No matter how fit you are, it only takes three to four weeks to become *un*conditioned. So if you have to stop exercising for one reason or another, don't feel bad that you cannot exercise at your previous level. Don't even try. Give your body a chance to rev up again.

WORKOUT

The keystone of my exercise program is my own Workout, which gives me the stretching I need to keep my muscles and ligaments (which link one bone to another) long and flexible. The exercises are rhythmic and sustained, so they provide cardiovascular conditioning. My Workout also includes exercises that are done against resistance, either that of my own body or ankle weights, so that I develop muscle tone.

I like having a routine that I can learn by heart and follow each day. This way I can compete with myself, keep track of how many repetitions I can do and see for myself to what extent my strength and endurance is increasing. Also, I do my Workout to music, which makes it more fun.

When you check out an exercise class, you should look for six things:

1. There should be a warm-up at the beginning of class. Warming up includes stretching and getting your pulse rate up. This helps your metabolic system get itself ready for the exercise which follows. The blood vessels in your muscles will expand and be prepared for receiving an increased flow of blood. The harder you work out—whether by jogging or some other form of aerobics, using machines or following a program of calisthenics—the more you should stretch, since heavily worked muscles tend to become shorter and more easily pulled.

2. There should be a cool-down at the end of class. Cooling down at the end of vigorous exercise is extremely important. While you exercise, an increased amount of blood is pumped to your heart with the help of contractions in the large leg muscles that press against the veins. If your leg muscles relax abruptly, the blood will collect in your extremities (athletes refer to this as "pooling") instead of getting back to your heart. Your heart is still pumping hard, but no blood is going up. When you slow down gradually, your muscles continue to assist in pumping up the blood until your pulse rate subsides, less blood is being pumped and your heart can handle it on its own.

During the cool-down, the muscles also are able to expel the toxic wastes produced by the metabolic process more easily.

3. The instructor's movements should be clear and precise so that you can follow them easily.

4. The instructor should demonstrate an understanding of the body and be concerned that students are doing each exercise correctly. You should be able to tell that she or he enjoys teaching and works to motivate each student to extend herself to her limits.

5. The exercise routine should be challenging.

6. When class is over you should stand straighter and feel exhilarated.

Whatever mode or combination of exercises you choose, it is always best to exercise on an empty stomach. After you eat, your heart pumps extra blood to your stomach to help in the digestive process. If you exercise on a full stomach, the blood will be diverted to the muscles, depriving the stomach of oxygen, which can result in cramps or nausea.

If you get thirsty during your workout, drink water. Afterwards, drink orange juice or some other natural fruit juice to replenish your supply of potassium and trace minerals. Do not drink soda pop. Why put something sugary or artificially sweetened, colored, flavored and carbonated into the body you've just worked so hard to make healthier?

You should not consider that you are through for the day once you have finished your jogging or your workout. The healthy woman will look for opportunities to continue using her body all day long. Here are a few exercise opportunities you can take advantage of. You will probably be able to add another six suggestions of your own.

1. Walk up a flight of stairs instead of taking the elevator or escalator.

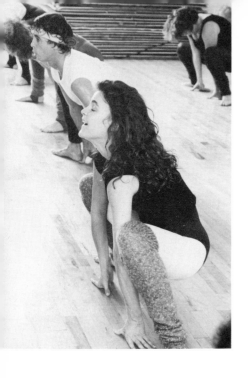

2. If you get a chance, stand with your toes on the edge of a step holding onto the railing or wall for support, and drop your heels as far below the step as you can. This gives you a good stretch in your calves.

3. Walk briskly to your nearby shopping center instead of driving.

4. When you bend or squat to pick something up, do it in a way that will give your hips and knees and hamstrings a stretch.

5. If you are standing and waiting, try rising up and down on your toes or tightening and releasing your buttocks muscles. You can do this while you are talking on the telephone too.

6. Stand up when you put on and take off your shoes and stockings to improve your balance.

Please remember that your goal is not to get pencil thin or to look like someone else. Your goal should be to take your body and make it as healthy, strong, flexible and well-proportioned as you can. Thin or plump, young or old, you will be more beautiful, have a prouder carriage, healthier glow and a supple flow of movement which says that you are comfortable and confident about your physical self.

A wonderful by-product of all these activities is that you will find new interests beginning to open up in your life.

Like me, you may never have thought of yourself as an athletic, outdoorsy sort of person. You were an observer. Sitting it out. Always a little too tired or worried that you wouldn't perform well enough. Group sports, camping trips, exploring one of our magnificent national parks was for *other* folks, probably of Scandinavian descent.

Since I started running and exercising regularly, I have developed a real desire to do these things. I *need* to be outside more. I seek clean air and natural beauty, and I'm always open to new activities because I have the stamina to do them. I don't want to be a bystander anymore. I want to participate, not necessarily to achieve excellence, but just to have fun.

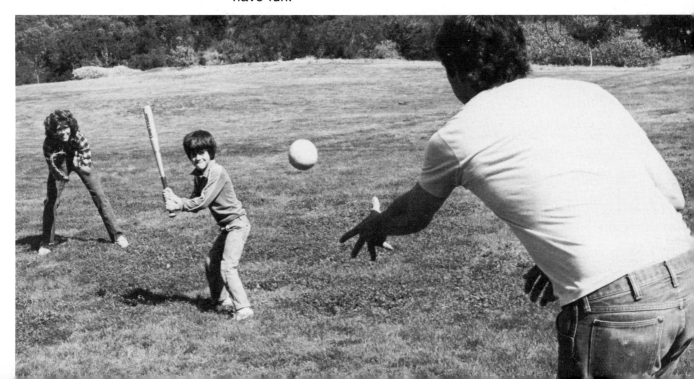

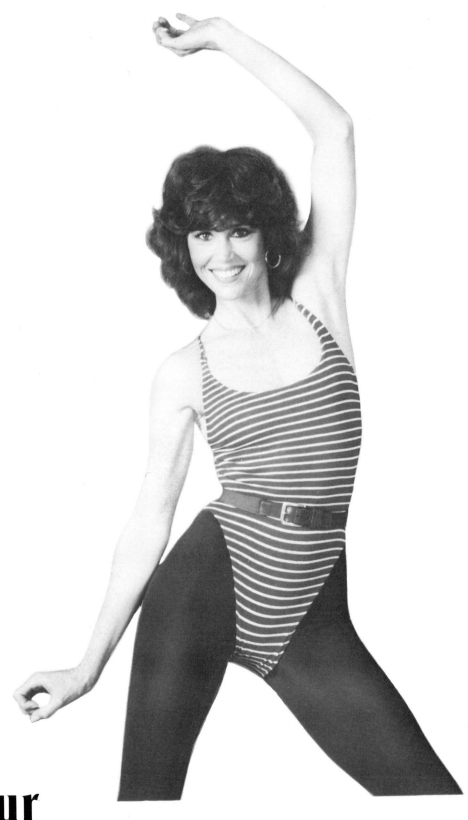

Part Four
The Workout

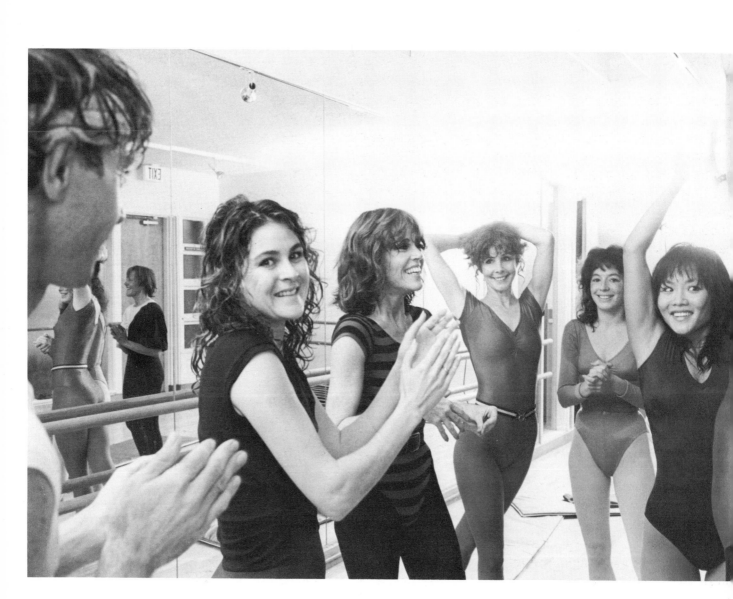

What It Is

It is a lot easier for most people—and I am one of them—to work out in a class or a gym. You have made the effort to get there, and you are there for one reason only. There are no distractions, and the teacher and the rest of the class are there to motivate you. You huff and you puff and you all hurt together and feel great together afterwards.

Sometimes it is too expensive to join a class or a gym, or there may not be a good one near where you live. You may travel a lot, or you may not have anyone to leave the children with. I can sympathize. These chapters are really for you. They give you everything you need for a good workout—except the time, the place and the commitment. You have to provide those yourself.

It means that you are going to have to be disciplined on your own, and you are going to have to find time to work out despite the telephone, the refrigerator, the children, the television set, a dirty house and all the rest. I have been there and I know it's hard. But it's worth it.

If you can find someone to work out with you, it will be easier. But whether you are alone or not, the first thing you must do is COMMIT YOURSELF TO DOING IT REGULARLY. You should work out to music at least three times a week with no interruptions.

MY WORKOUT PROGRAM

The exercises that follow are basically the ones I do myself. I did not invent them, but I have worked with them, modified them and placed them in a sequence that works for me and for the people who come to my Workout Studios. They are designed to build strength, develop flexibility and increase endurance. And there is no question that this exercise program can alter the shape of your body, burn away those fatty deposits and develop muscle tone where you never knew you could have any. It will make you feel good, physically and psychologically. But you must commit yourself to regular, vigorous exercise, eat properly and get enough sleep.

The exercises are carefully structured to use each part of the body in a specific sequence. You may be tempted to go straight to the ones that attack your trouble spots. This is all right once in a great while when you are short of time, but it is really missing the point of the workout. An effective workout requires the vigorous and sustained use of your entire body for at least 20 to 40 minutes. This will not only tone muscles in a specific area, but burn up calories, improve your circulation, eliminate toxins, and strengthen your heart and lungs.

The basis of the Workout is the repetition of certain movements that use a single muscle group against the resistance of your own body weight. We work each muscle group to its maximum. The repetitions are followed by stretches to develop flexibility and to keep your muscles long. The stretches are every bit as important as the repetitions.

THE BURN

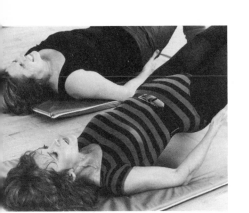

From this point on, I will often mention the "burn" and exhort you to "go for the burn." This burn is a unique sensation that you get when you have used a muscle very strenuously. You feel the burn and you find that you have difficulty contracting that muscle for a moment. Newcomers to exercise often worry about it, but don't be concerned; it is simply a sign that you are exercising that particular muscle vigorously and effectively, working hard and deep.

The burn is the result of a chemical reaction in your body. During the normal metabolic process, the carbohydrate fuel in your muscle is converted to a chemical known as pyruvate. Pyruvate combines with oxygen and then the combination breaks down into carbon dioxide and water which is carried away in the blood and expelled from the body as waste gases.

If there is not enough oxygen available to combine with the pyruvate, the pyruvate turns into lactic acid, which is a toxin. The build-up of lactic acid is what causes the burning sensation and impedes muscle contraction.

There is absolutely nothing harmful or dangerous about it. It just slows you down until the oxygen supply is replenished, which is a matter of seconds. Once there is enough oxygen again, the lactic acid converts back into pyruvate.

If you are very fit, you will be able to exercise longer before you feel that burn than someone who is out of shape. When I first did the buttocks exercise described on pages 124–126, my muscles burned so much I had to stop three or four times during the exercise. Now the burn comes later and I don't have to stop. I've even come to look forward to it. It lets me know that I'm really working hard.

WEIGHTS

For most of you the weight of your body will provide sufficient resistance during the repetitions, but by the time you have worked up to the advanced exercises, or if you are already accustomed to exercise, you may find that your muscles have grown used to your body weight. If you can get through the advanced Workout fairly easily without feeling the burn, then instead of increasing the number of repetitions, you should add ankle weights.

A muscle is composed of fibers—the larger the muscle, the more bers it contains. To get the full use of your muscle, all the fibers should be called into action. But your muscle will only use the number of fibers that it really needs. At first it will take all the fibers in your abdominal muscles to lift your legs up when you are on your back, but when these muscles get stronger, they will only need to use a fraction of their fibers. And that is all they will use, no matter how many leg lifts you do. This means it is time to add weights.

You can buy two-and-a-half-pound weights, which are what most of my students start with, at most sporting goods stores. They go on at the beginning of the abdominal exercises and stay on for the rest of the class.

You will not be able to do all the repetitions at first when you are wearing weights. That is all right. Do as many as you can before your muscles give out, and then go on to the next exercise. It is better to use all of a muscle for a short time than to do a hundred repetitions using only part of it.

If you are worried about developing bulging muscles, don't be. Women—99.9 percent of us—do not have enough testosterone, the male hormone that governs muscle growth, to develop bulgy muscles. But something muscle-like does happen and I like it. Since you are reading this book, you are probably like me and appreciate a woman's body on which the muscle cuts and contours are evident. This is what you will get with regular workouts.

PREPARING FOR YOUR WORKOUT

1. Try to set a regular time to exercise. I prefer working out early in the morning. I get it out of the way and start the day with high energy. You may find it easier after work when you've been sitting all day and the tension has built up. Or the afternoon, when the baby is sleeping, may be best for you.

Exercise in the early evening can relax you, relieve tension and help keep you from overeating at dinner. In the afternoon, it can serve as a pick-me-up and revitalize you for the rest of the day. Choose the time that suits your schedule best and then stick to it. Getting a routine going is half the battle. But don't feel you have failed if you miss a workout for some good reason. The guilt will make you feel discouraged and that old self-punishment syndrome—eating—might set in.

2. Turn the phone off before you start.

3. You need a place to exercise where there is no draft and the ceiling is high enough to allow you to jump up and clap your hands overhead. You need room enough to swing your arms wide without hitting anything.

4. You need an exercise pad or towel or blanket to give you a little padding for your floor work. If you are on a carpet, put a towel under you to delineate your workout space and keep the dust and fibers out of your nose and hair.

5. Dress for it. An exercise outfit helps because it sets this time apart from the rest of your day and makes it matter more. I prefer a leotard and tights. If I'm feeling overweight, I put on a pair of those baggy "sweat" pants that feel like parachute silk with an elastic belt. They cover up a multitude of sins and help heat your body faster. I always wear leg warmers to keep my leg muscles warm—and because they make me feel like a dancer. You should feel comfortable and be able to move freely.

6. A big mirror to exercise in front of makes it a lot easier. Count yourself lucky if you have one. If not, it is not an essential.

MUSIC

My experience has been that exercising with music is easier and more fun than without it. It helps carry you through the pain. I cannot even conceive of doing my workout without music.

I have made tapes of both the beginner and advanced classes. I call out the instructions and count the repetitions to music. When I travel and can't carry records or there's no stereo, I just bring my tape and a small tape recorder and I'm all set. *

Each section of the Workout uses different music. I have suggested songs that we like using at the Workout Studio. Use them as a guide to the rhythm you will need. You may prefer other songs, but try to use music with the right rhythm, a steady easy-to-follow beat, and with a long enough running time so you won't have to get up and start it over more than once. Experiment a little. Make the music an important part of your routine. I normally do not care for disco, but I have found it is great to exercise to because of the steady driving beat and because the songs are long. As you can see from my suggestions with each group of exercises, I use a little of everything from Pop to Country and Western and Rock.

HOW TO DO IT

In the beginning, it will seem very mechanical. You will be trying to read the instructions and figure out when to breathe while trying all these new positions. Do not rush it. Read the instructions carefully. It is important that you do the exercises correctly, otherwise you risk getting

*Perform these exercises to music by The Jacksons, REO Speedwagon, Brothers Johnson and many more on my Workout Record and Workout Tape, available on the CBS label in all good department stores and record shops in the UK.

hurt. And you won't be getting as much as you should from your efforts.

Memorize the exercise series as quickly as possible and then put the book away. The exercises are designed to flow from one to the next without stopping, which is hard to do when you are following a book. So read and re-read each section several times and go through the motions slowly to become familiar with them before you start with the music. It takes more time at the beginning, but it is worth it for the enjoyment you will have in moving from one section to the next.

Once you have reached this point, here is what you should do to have the most fun and get the most out of your workout.

1. Turn on the music you have chosen for the section, get in the correct starting position and—begin!

2. Go from exercise one to exercise two, and on and on without stopping until you have finished that section.

3. Stop.

4. Change the music and go on to the next section.

5. Do the exercises in the order indicated. They are designed to be done in sequence, one after the other. If no starting position is given, it means that the exercise begins in the same position where the one before it ended.

6. Maintain the momentum. This is extremely important. If you stop to answer the phone or whatever, your muscles will cool down. Cold muscles tear and sustain injury more easily. The cardiovascular benefits are lessened if your effort is not sustained. And psychologically, it is harder to start up again once you stop.

BEGINNER OR ADVANCED?

You should start with the beginners' class unless you have had considerable exercise experience. Once you can do the beginners' workout all the way through smoothly and without strain, move up to the advanced class and gradually increase the number of repetitions to the amount indicated. Once you can do all the repetitions without strain, add the weights.

Do what you can. Don't push yourself too hard or you may get hurt. On the other hand, if it is easy, it is not going to be effective. You have to challenge your body. Make yourself sweat. You always have to push a little beyond what you think you can do. You will be surprised at the untapped reserves of energy and strength you did not know you had.

When you think you can't do any more repetitions, do two more! Go for the burn! Sweat!

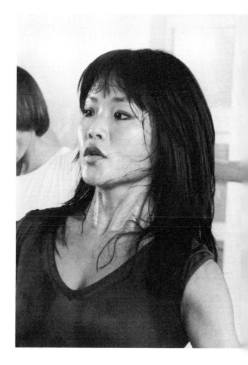

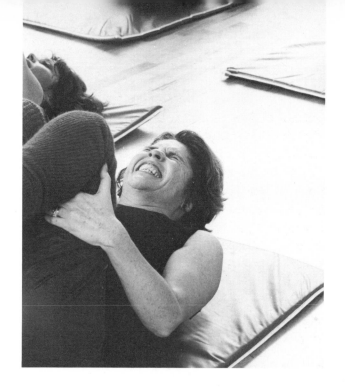

PAIN

There is a natural healthy pain that comes with any major exertion. The burn I talk about is that kind of pain. There is also the pain that tells you something is wrong. Learn to listen to your body. It will tell you when there is a problem. And learn to read your pain. If something seems wrong, stop immediately and try to understand what it is. If it persists, I recommend you see a good chiropractor.

BREATHING

The function of the lungs is to draw oxygen in and send it into the bloodstream, and to expel carbon dioxide from our bodies. By this process our blood is cleansed of toxins and the cells of our body are repaired and energized. I indicate the proper breathing in each exercise. It is important to inhale and exhale as indicated. You may find that you have a tendency to hold your breath. Don't. You need to get that oxygen into your bloodstream. And you need to breathe out to eliminate waste products and toxic gases. In general, you should breathe out when you are making the most effort and breathe in when you ease up.

TIPS

1. Newcomers to exercise may experience—as I did—muscle swelling. You will be looking forward to a looser fit in your slacks and to your horror you find they are tighter. Not to worry. You are working your muscles hard. It is as if someone punched them. They swell, but the swelling goes down very rapidly.

2. Pay more attention to losing inches than to losing pounds. Muscle weighs more than fat, so as you build strength your weight may stay the same or even increase slightly. But you will lose inches and your proportions will change for the better. To lose weight, you must cut back on your calories.

3. You will be stiff at first. You can minimize this by hopping into a hot bath after your workout before your muscles have cooled down. But do your exercises even if you are stiff. This will help dissipate the stiffness, and you will be surprised how quickly your muscles adapt as you maintain your routine. After the first week or so, you will probably not feel stiff any more.

4. I've said it before, but I'll say it again because it's important. Never eat before exercising. It might nauseate you. Your blood will be diverted to help in the digestive process just when it is needed to carry oxygen to your muscles.

5. Always remember to empty your bladder before starting.

AND FINALLY . . .

It takes work and time. You are about to begin something that I hope will become a permanent part of your life. It is important to understand that you will only get out of it what you put into it. Toning and firming can begin to show within days, but for a deep, total and lasting effect, you need to work hard and regularly. If you do, you will find as I have that the rewards are immeasurable.

AND ONE MORE THING . . .

I want you to know who the models are in the photographs that accompany the exercises. They are all very special. I have told you about Janice. Then there is Debra Feuer, who is a dancer. And Carol Gutierrez, who is also a dancer. Carol teaches at the Workout Studio and is in charge of teacher training there. And there is Jennifer Parsons, also a dancer.

And there is one model whom I'm extra fond of—my stepmother, Shirlee Fonda, who introduced me to that first great exercise class that got me started on all this. Take a look at Shirlee, who works out every day, and I think you'll join me in saying, "Let's hear it for forty-five and over." Do you need anything more to convince you of the benefits of regular, vigorous exercise?

IT'S TIME TO GET STARTED.

CONCENTRATE ON WHAT YOU ARE DOING

NO DISTRACTIONS
CENTER YOURSELF
THIS IS *YOUR* TIME

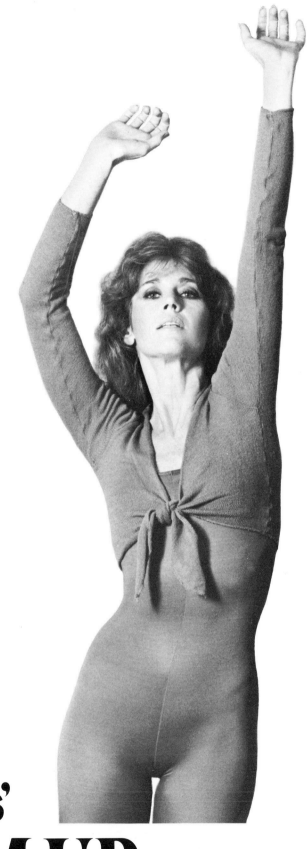

Beginners' WARM-UP

WARM-UP 5 MINUTES

Purpose: To increase the pulse rate, heat up and stretch out the muscles in every part of the body. No exercise session should begin without warming up. Cold muscles are more easily injured.

Music:

London Symphony Orchestra—"Theme from *Star Wars*"/*Star Wars*
Donna Summer—"Fairy Tale High"/*Live and More*
Irene Cara—"Red Light"/*Fame*
Kongas—"Gimme Some Lovin' "/*Africanism*
Barbra Streisand—"Main Event"/*Main Event*

One

HEAD ROLLS

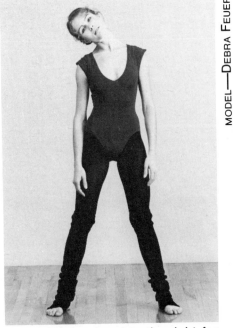 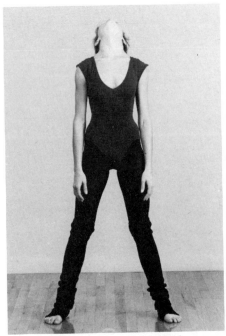

MODEL—DEBRA FEUER

Starting position: Standing, place feet a little more than hip distance apart. Pull up out of the torso, stomach pulled in, buttocks squeezed tight, shoulders down, arms at sides.

1. Rotate your head to the right for one count. Feel the stretch up the left side of your neck. Don't let your shoulders hunch up.

2. Rotate your head back for one count. Stretch your chin to the ceiling and let your mouth open.

76

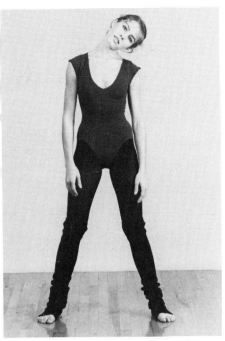 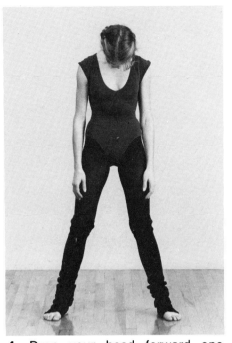

3. Rotate your head to the left one count.

4. Drop your head forward one count, stretching your chin to your chest. Feel the pull up the back of your neck.

Repeat the same movement to the right, again taking one count for each position. Then reverse and do the same thing two times to the left.

Breathing: Normal

Two SHOULDER LIFTS

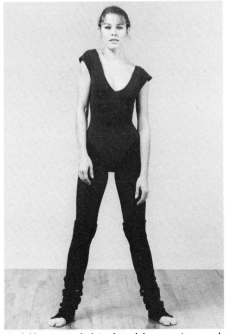 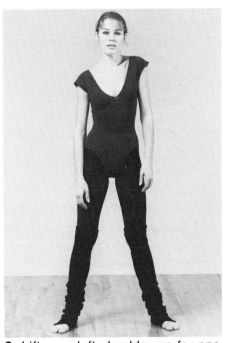

1. Lift your right shoulder up toward your ear for one count.

2. Lift your left shoulder up for one count as you lower your right shoulder.

Repeat right and left shoulder lifts for a total of 8 counts.

Breathing: Normal

Three SIDE STRETCHES

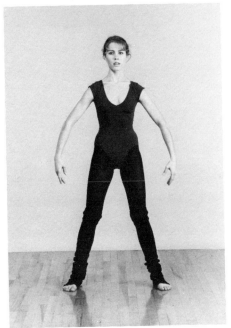

1. Inhale as you open your arms to the side.

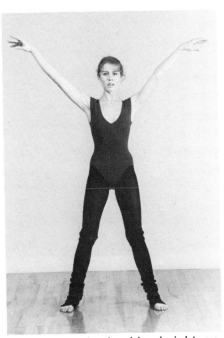

As they reach shoulder height exhale . . .

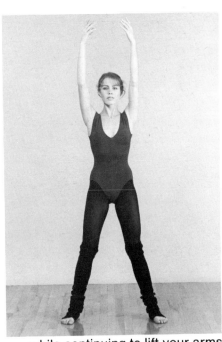

. . . while continuing to lift your arms over your head.

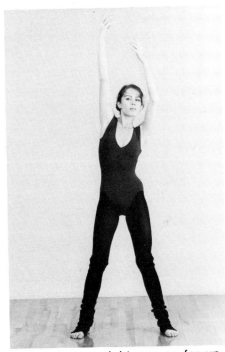

2. Reach your right arm as far upward toward the ceiling as you can for one count. Feel the stretch up your right side.

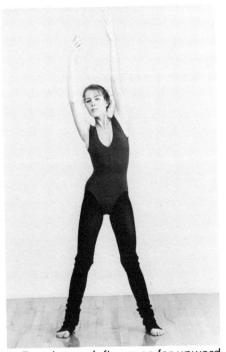

3. Reach your left arm as far upward as you can for one count. Feel the stretch up your left side.

Repeat, reaching right and left, for a total of 8 counts.

Breathing: Normal

Four
WAIST REACHES

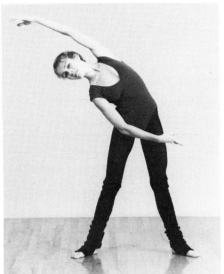 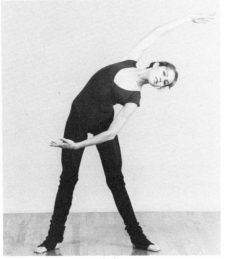

1. Pulling outward and directly to the side, reach your left arm over your head to the right. Gently bounce for 4 counts, keeping hips forward, left shoulder back, and right arm curved in front of you.

2. Reach your right arm over your head to the left and bounce for 4 counts, curving your left arm in front of you.

Repeat once to the right and to the left.

Breathing: Normal

Five
HAMSTRING STRETCHES

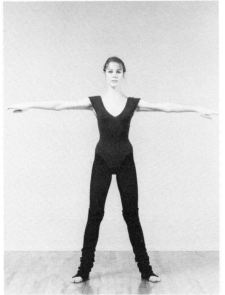 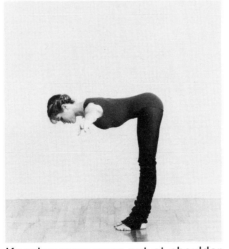

Starting position: When you complete the final reach to the left in the previous exercise come back to center position, opening your arms to shoulder height for 2 counts while you inhale.

Keeping your arms out at shoulder height take 4 counts to bend forward with a flat back and straight legs. Exhale as you bend forward. Stretch your chin outward, your buttocks to the ceiling and "pulse" the small of your back downward in little bounces for a count of 8.

Breathing: Normal

Six

HAMSTRING STRETCHES

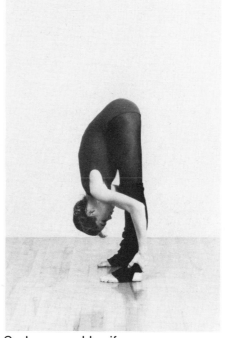

Grab your ankles if you can, or your calves, and pull down for 8 counts.

Breathing: Normal; careful not to hold your breath.

Seven

SPINE STRETCH

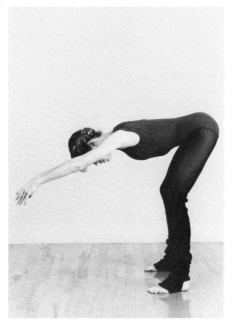

Starting position: Raise torso so it is parallel to floor, arms stretched out, knees bent.

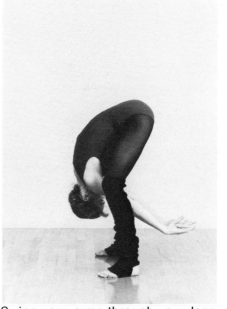

Swing your arms through your legs and return to starting position 8 times. Take one count for each swing through and return.

Breathing: Exhale as you swing through legs. Inhale as you come up to starting position.

Eight
HAMSTRING STRETCHES

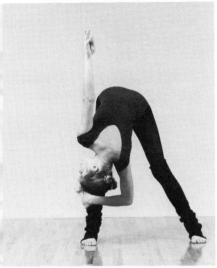 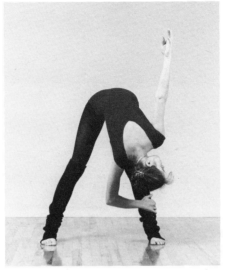 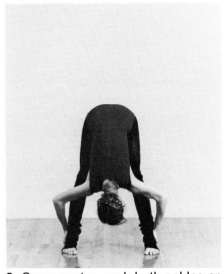

1. Straighten your legs again, grab your right ankle or calf with your left hand and pull your torso down over your right leg. Let your right arm reach up toward the ceiling. Pull down this way, thinking of stretching your chest to your knee, for 4 counts.

2. Repeat the same movement to the left side for 4 counts, grabbing your left ankle or calf with your right hand and letting your left arm reach upward.

Repeat for a total of 4 counts right, 4 counts left.

3. Come center, grab both ankles or calves and pull down 4 counts.

Breathing: Steady breathing

Nine
HAMSTRING STRETCHES

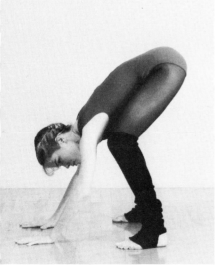 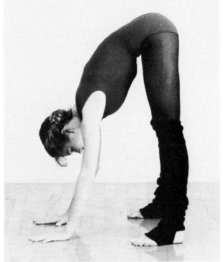

Starting position: Bend your knees, feet apart, and place your hands on the floor in front of you.

Straighten and bend your knees trying to keep your hands on the floor. The two movements—bending and straightening—are done to one count. Do this for 8 counts.

Breathing: Exhale as you straighten, inhale as you bend.

Ten

CALF RAISES

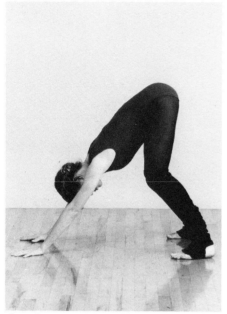

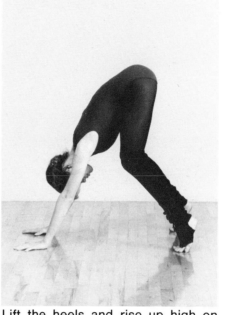

Do this 20 times. Go for the burn!

Breathing: Exhale as you rise up on toes, inhale as you lower heels.

Starting position: Keep your feet apart, bend your knees slightly and walk your hands away from your body.

Lift the heels and rise up high on your toes, as high as you possibly can to really work your ankles and calves, then lower your heels again.

Eleven INNER THIGH STRETCH

Starting position: Walk your hands back in between the legs, bend your knees into a squatting position and place your hands behind your feet. You'll find your inner knees are resting on your elbows, which should stretch your inner thighs open.

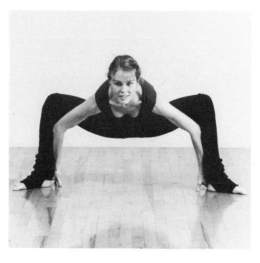

Small bounces with your buttocks for 16 counts.

Breathing: Normal

Twelve ROLL-UP

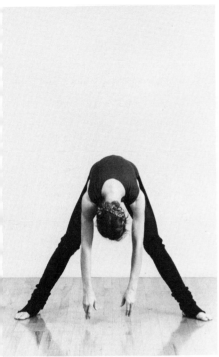 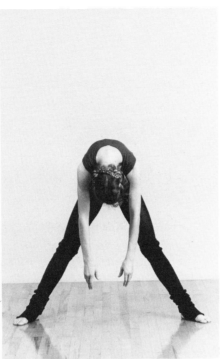 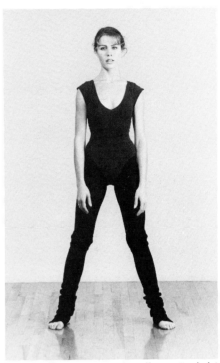

Starting position: Let go of your feet, straighten your knees, let your arms and head hang limp like a rag doll.

Slowly roll up, one vertebra at a time,

. . . until you are standing straight and erect, exactly as you began the warm-up.

Breathing: Normal

Thirteen

Purpose:

This aerobic section is part of the warm-up. Now that you have begun to limber up and get the blood flowing, you will further increase your pulse rate, burn up some calories and begin to strengthen your heart and lungs. It will be difficult at first, but hang in there. Before long it will seem easy and as you build cardiovascular strength you will feel tremendous exhilaration and increased energy.

It is crucial that you remember to breathe deeply and regularly all during these aerobic exercises. As the heart is called upon to pump blood faster to your muscles, your lungs must send larger amounts of oxygen into the bloodstream to be carried to the muscles and to carry away the waste gases.

Music:

Continue with the same music used in the beginning of the warm-up.

Starting position: Standing erect, feet together, pull up out of the torso.

MODEL—CAROL GUTIERREZ

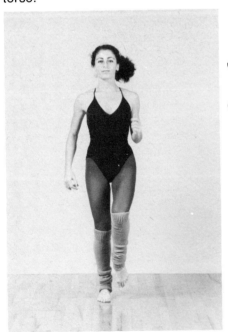

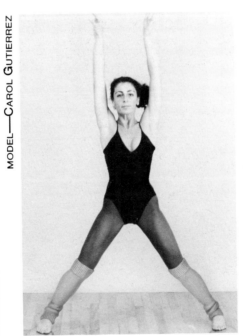

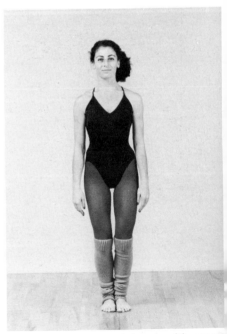

1. Jog in place for 20 counts. On each count both the right and left feet touch down. You should land on the balls of your feet and then work through the whole foot, being sure to let the heels touch down.

2. Jumping jacks for 10 counts: Jump up and open your legs, landing with your legs apart as your arms swing out to the side and up over your head.

Then jump up and land with your feet together as you bring your arms down to your sides again. These two jumps are done to one count.

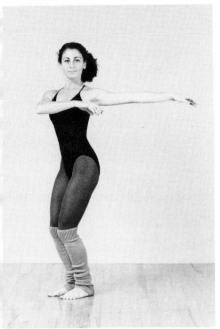

3. Jumping twists for 10 counts: Jump and twist your body to the right as you swing your arms to the left, . . .

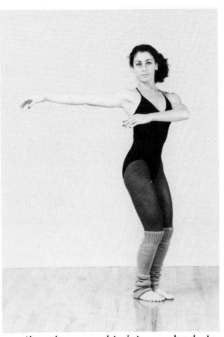

. . . then jump and twist your body to the left swinging your arms to the right. These two movements are done to one count.

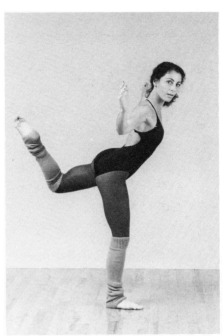

4. Heels up, knees up: Jog in place for 5 counts, lifting your heels up behind you.

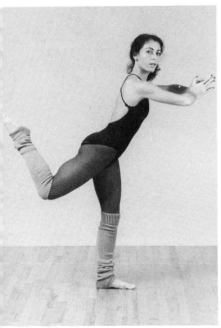

On each count both the right and left heels lift up.

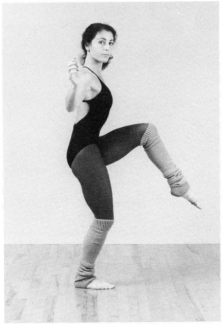

Then, while you continue jogging in place, prance for 5 counts, lifting your knees high in front of you.

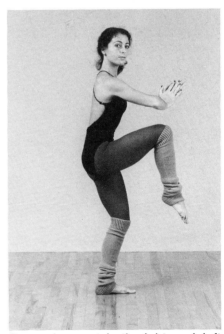

On each count both right and left knees lift. Clap your hands when the right leg lifts on each count.

CONTINUED→

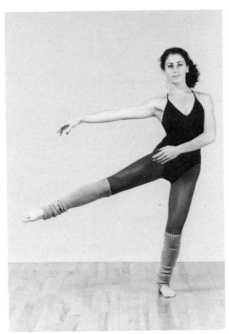

5. Leg swings for 10 counts: Jump, landing on your left foot, and swing your right leg and your arms out to the right side.

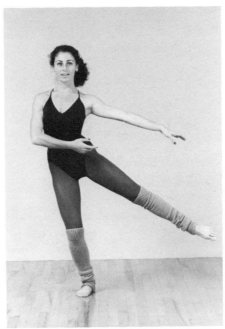

Repeat to the left. These two jumps are done to one count.

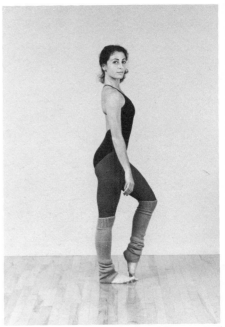

6. Jog in place again for 10 counts, slowing down until only your heels are lifting off the floor, to allow the pulse rate to gradually slow down.

Fourteen

ROLL-DOWN AND KNEE BENDS

Starting position: Feet together, arms hanging at your sides, stomach pulled in, buttocks tight.

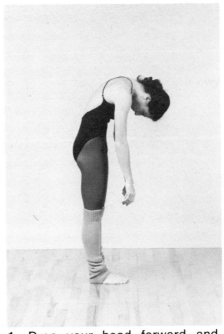

1. Drop your head forward and, keeping knees straight, roll down the spine, one vertebra at a time. Let your arms hang limp like a rag doll.

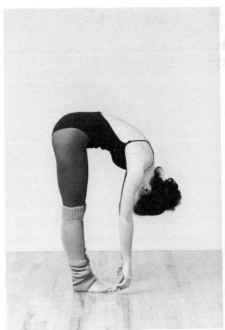

Take 4 counts for hands to touch the floor.

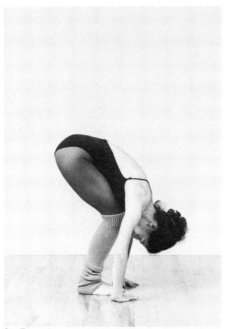

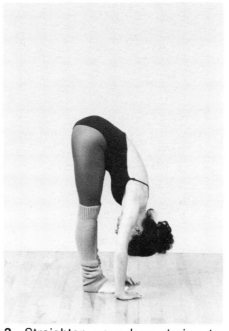

Breathing: Exhale as you straighten your knees. Inhale as you bend them.

2. Bend your knees and place your hands on the floor.

3. Straighten your legs, trying to keep your hands on the floor. Bend and straighten to one count. Do this for 8 counts.

Fifteen

TENDON STRETCH

Starting position: Still bending forward from the hip, walk your hands way out in front of you. Straighten both legs.

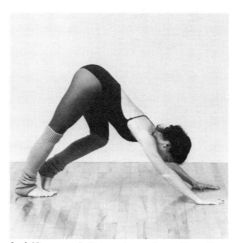

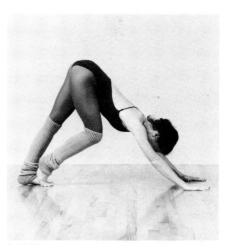

1. Lift your left heel up, bending the left knee, while you bounce your right heel to the floor for 4 counts.

2. Lift your right heel up, bending the right knee and straightening the left, while you bounce your left heel to the floor for 4 counts.

Repeat 3 times to each side, alternating right and left.

Breathing: Normal

Sixteen

ROLL-UP AND STRETCH

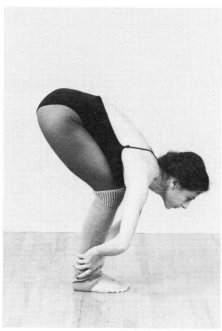

Starting position: Walk your hands back to your legs, bend your knees, feet together.

1. Grab your ankles or calves, keeping your knees bent.

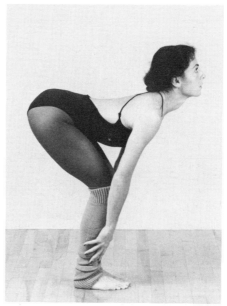

2. Arch your back, lifting your head and chin up for 4 counts. Then reach out with your chest even farther, arching your back as much as you can and reaching your buttocks toward the ceiling for 4 counts.

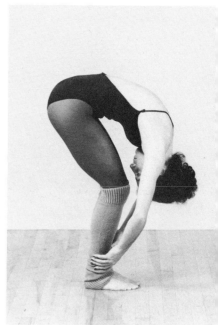

3. Round your back, pull down torso over your thighs.

Repeat movements 1, 2 and 3 once

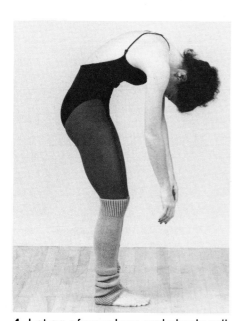

4. Let go of your legs and slowly roll up, one vertebra at a time.

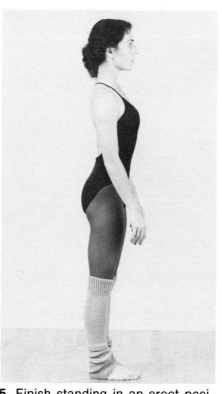

5. Finish standing in an erect position, stomach pulled in, buttocks tight, pulling up out of your torso.

Breathing: Inhale, then exhale as you arch up; inhale, then exhale as you round down.

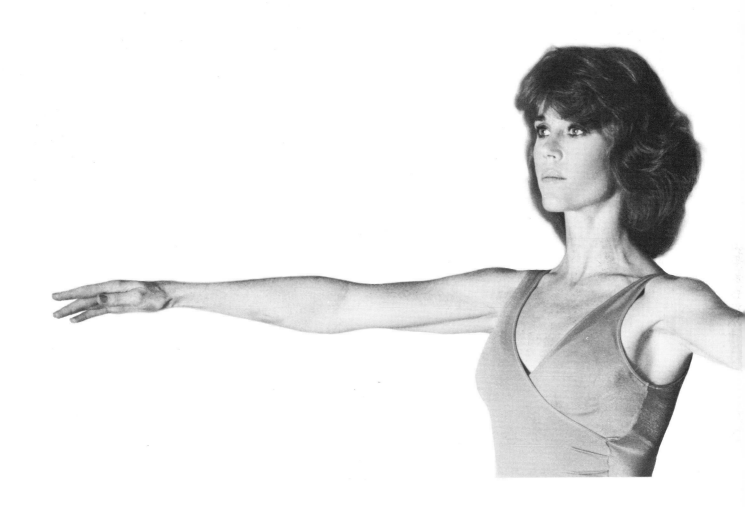

Beginners'
ARMS

ARMS 4 MINUTES

Purpose:
To strengthen, tone and render flexible every part of your arms, shoulders and chest.

Music:
Irene Cara—"Fame"/*Fame*
Irene Cara—"Red Light"/*Fame*
Kongas—"Gimme Some Lovin' "/*Africanism*
Karen Young—"Hot Shot"/*Hot Shot*
Dan Hartman—"Instant Replay"/*Instant Replay*
Paul Jabara—"Pleasure Island"/*Keeping Time*
Johnny Lee—"Lookin' for Love"/*Urban Cowboy*

One   STRAIGHT ARM CIRCLES
Deltoids, trapezius

Starting position: Stand with feet together, buttocks tight, stomach pulled in, body pulled up, shoulders down.

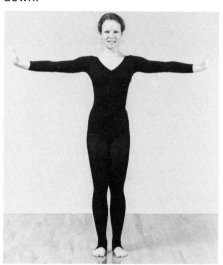 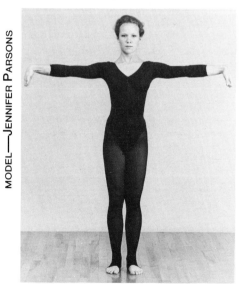 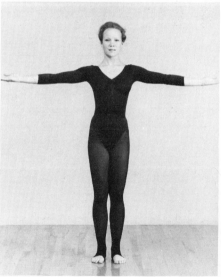

MODEL—JENNIFER PARSONS

1. Arms straight out to the side with wrists flexed upward, heels of your hands pushing to opposite walls. Circle the arms forward 8 counts and back 8 counts, being sure to keep the shoulders from hunching up. The circling motion is with the entire arm from the shoulder. Make the circles as large as you can.

2. Repeat circling 8 counts forward, 8 counts back, with wrists flexed downward, backs of hands pushing to side walls as hard as you can, knuckles folded under.

3. Repeat circling 8 counts forward, 8 counts back with palms facing the ceiling.

Breathing: Steady breathing

90

Two

SHOULDER RELEASE
Deltoids

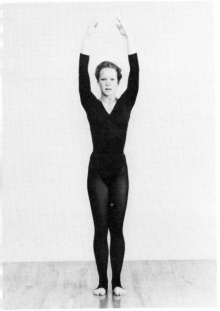

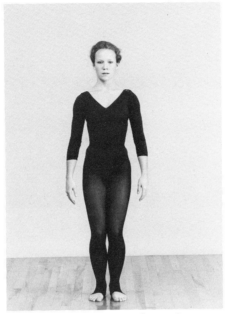

Starting position: Bring your arms down to your sides.

1. Swing your arms out to the side and over your head.

2. Swing your arms down to your sides as you bend your knees slightly.

These two movements are done to one count. Do a total of 8 counts, straightening the knees as you repeat movement 1.

Breathing: Exhale as arms come down. Inhale as arms go up.

Three

ELBOW EXTENSIONS
Triceps

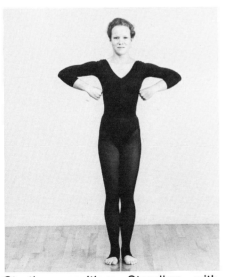

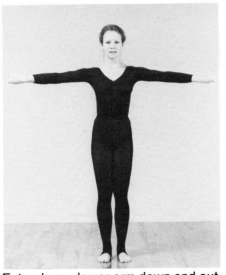

Starting position: Standing with knees straight, raise your elbows out to the side at shoulder height. Your lower arm is bent in toward your body, fists are clenched, palms facing back wall.

Extend your lower arm down and out to shoulder height. Try not to move your shoulders or upper arms, and keep your palms facing behind you, fists clenched.

Return to starting position. Open and close your lower arms like this 10 times.

Breathing: Exhale as you extend arm from elbow. Inhale as you bring lower arm back to starting position.

Four

SHOULDER TWISTS
Deltoids, triceps

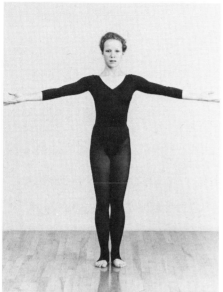

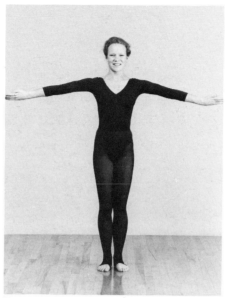

Starting position: Arms are extended straight to the side, shoulder height, palms up.

Rotate your arms forward from the shoulders, then release your arms backward from the shoulder to starting position.

The two movements are done to one count. Do for 16 counts. Imagine you're turning a doorknob with each hand.

Be sure not to move anything but your arms. It's a small movement which should cause a burning sensation. Good! Go for it!

Breathing: Exhale as arm turns forward from shoulder. Inhale as arm releases back.

Five

SHOULDER RELEASE
Deltoids

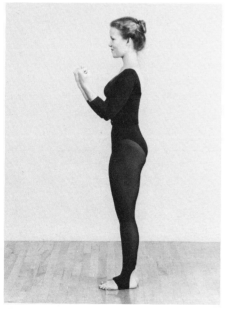

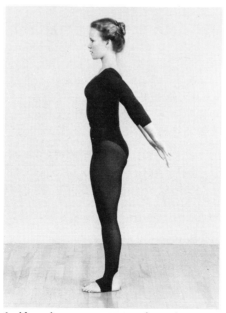

Starting position: Bring your arms in front of you, parallel to each other with elbows bent, fists clenched.

1. Keeping your arms close to your sides, swing them down and behind you as far as you can without moving your torso. The hands open, palms to back wall, at the end of the swing.

2. Then pull arms forward to starting position.

The swing back and pull forward are done to one count. Repeat for total of 8 counts.

Breathing: Exhale as arms swing behind body. Inhale as arms pull forward.

Six

BACK OF THE ARM EXTENSIONS
Triceps

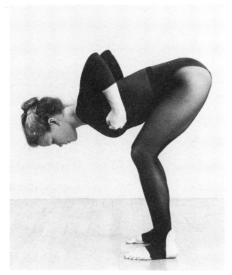

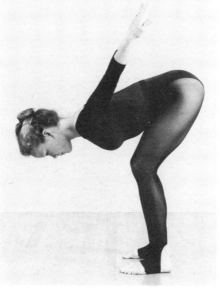

2. Then bend arms in again as in starting position.

These two movements are done to one count. Repeat for a total of 10 counts. Be sure to keep arms close to your sides.

Breathing: Exhale as arms extend behind body. Inhale as arms bend in.

Starting position: Place your feet a little more than hip distance apart. Bend your knees and bend forward keeping your back flat, your elbows bent, arms close to your sides, your fists held at the sides of your breasts.

1. Keeping your knees bent, extend your arms and hands straight up as high as possible behind your back, opening your hands, fingers stretching out.

Seven

PULLING WEEDS
Biceps

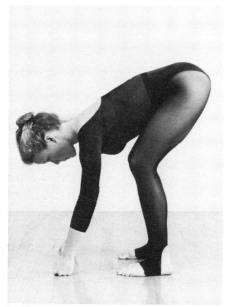

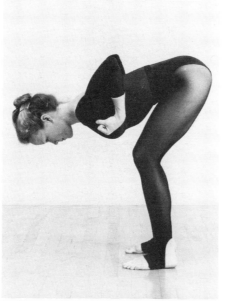

These two movements are done to one count. Repeat for a total of 10 counts.

Breathing: Exhale as you pull arms up. Inhale as you reach forward.

1. Keeping your knees bent, reach forward with your arms as though you were grabbing weeds.

2. Now quickly pull your arms back with your elbows bent behind you, fists clenched, as though you were angrily pulling up the weeds.

Eight SCISSORS
Pectorals

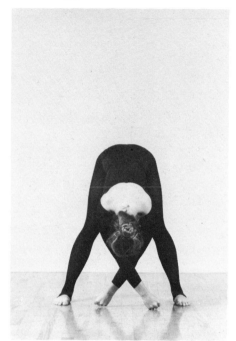

Starting position: Standing with feet a little more than hip distance apart, let your body hang over with arms crossed.

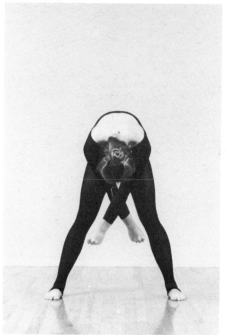

1. As you roll up through the spine, cross the left arm over the right arm, then the right arm over the left arm, in a scissoring motion.

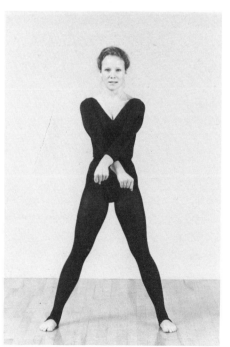

2. When you've rolled up to a standing position, continue to scissor the arms upward.

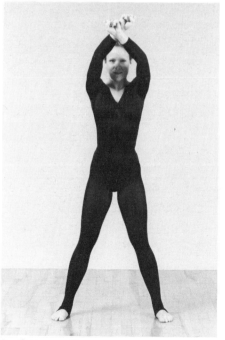

3. Scissor the arms up over your head then scissor them back down again, as you remain standing up straight.

Take 8 counts to bring the arms up and 8 counts to bring them down.

Try to open the arms as wide as you can before you scissor them and try not to move the rest of the body. This is an excellent exercise for the pectoral muscles, which hold up the breasts.

Breathing: Steady breathing

Nine

ARM STRETCHES
Pectorals

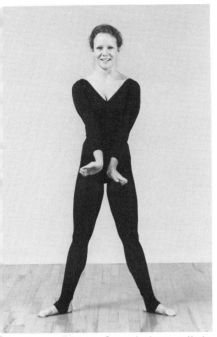

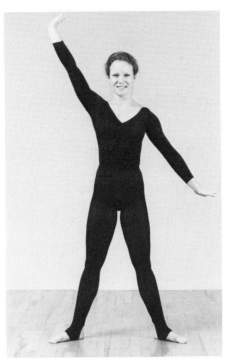

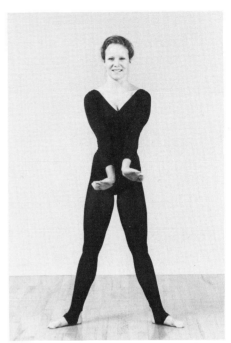

Starting position: Stand, feet a little wider than hip distance apart, with arms straight and held in front of you, both hands flexed, knuckles folded under.

1. Swing your right arm diagonally up and back over your head, while your left arm swings diagonally down and back, opening your chest in a diagonal pull.

2. Bring arms together as in starting position. These two movements are done to one count. Repeat movements 1 and 2 (*i.e.,* do this for 2 counts to the right).

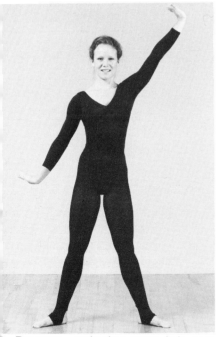

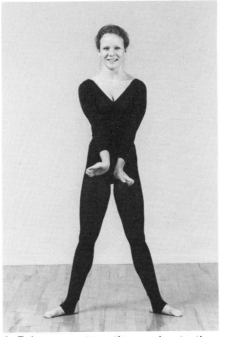

3. Reverse, swinging your left arm up and your right arm down and back.

4. Bring arms together as in starting position. These two movements are done to one count. Repeat movements 3 and 4 (*i.e.,* do for 2 counts to the left).

Do the entire set twice, a total of 8 counts.

Breathing: Exhale as both arms move out. Inhale as they meet in front of you.

SHAKE YOUR ARMS OUT.

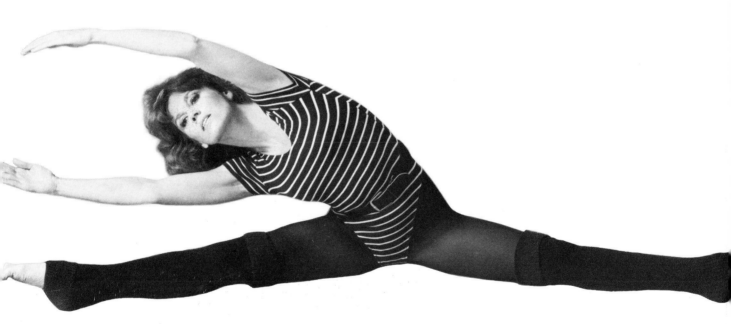

Beginners'
WAIST

WAIST 5 MINUTES (including floor work)

Purpose:
To reduce the fatty deposits at the waistline, tone, shape and strengthen th waist and back muscles.

Music:

Jacksons—"Can You Feel It"/ *Triumph*
Roberta Kelly—"Oh Happy Day"/ *Gettin' the Spirit*
Roberta Kelly—"To My Father's House"/ *Gettin' the Spirit*
Isaac Hayes—"Don't Let Go"/ *Don't Let Go*
Eddie Rabbitt—"I Love a Rainy Night"/ *Horizon*
Donna Summer—"Hot Stuff"/ *Bad Girls*
Donna Summer—"MacArthur Park"/ *Live and More*
Pattie Brooks—"Don't Make Me Wait"/ *Love Shook*
Amii Stewart—"Light My Fire"/ *Knock on Wood*

One

SIDE PULLS
Intercostals, obliques

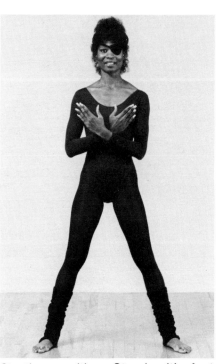 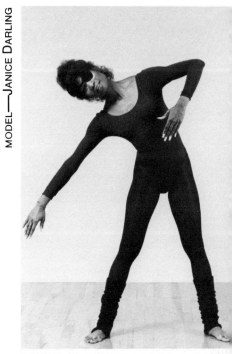

MODEL—JANICE DARLING

Starting position: Stand with feet apart, stomach pulled in, buttocks tight, hands in front of your torso, palms facing your body. Imagine you are standing between two sheets of glass. If you lean forward you'll break the glass.

1. Pull over to the right, reachin down and out with your right arr while your left elbow bends upwar as far as it can go. You should feel pull up the left side of your body. Le your head relax to the right. Kee your left shoulder back and you hips forward.

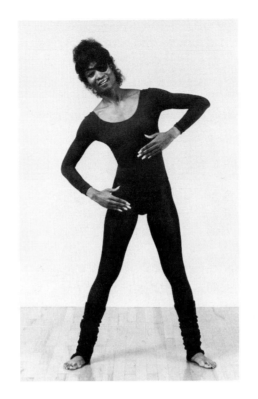

ome back up toward the starting
osition before reaching out again.
his down and up movement is done
 one count. Do 20 counts to the
ght.

2. Repeat 20 counts to the left, reaching down with your left arm and up with your bent right elbow. Be sure to keep your right shoulder back and your hips forward.

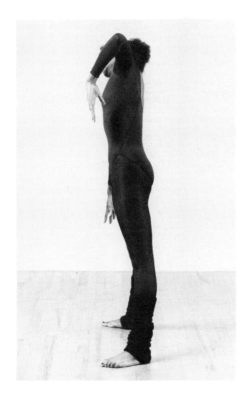

his is probably the most effective
xercise I've found for slimming the
aist, but in order to get the most
ut of it you must go directly to the
de and not let your upper torso pull
rward.

Breathing: Exhale as you reach out. Inhale as you come up between reaches.

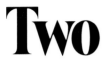

MORE SIDE PULLS
Intercostals, obliques

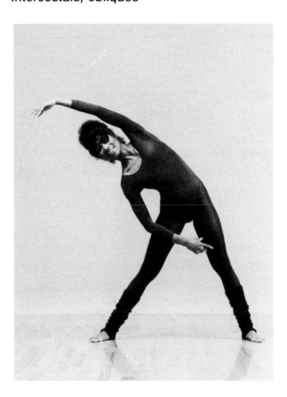

1. Pull over to the right, extendin[g] your left arm directly over your ea[r] your right arm curved in front of yo[u] Bounce gently for 8 counts, bein[g] sure to keep your hips forwar[d] weight evenly distributed on bo[th] feet, and left shoulder back.

2. Place both hands behind your head and bounce gently to the right side for 8 counts. Don't let your elbows pull inward; keep them opened outward.

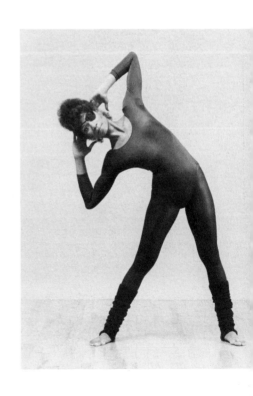

Reach both arms to the right, grab your left wrist with your right hand and pull over, pulsing gently for 8 counts.

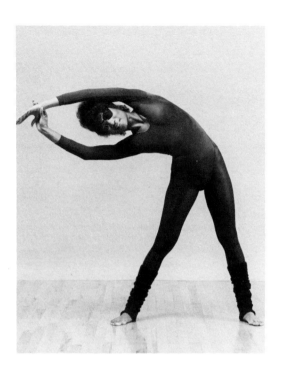

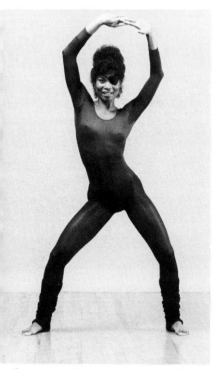

. Come back to the center, bend our knees, clasp hands and circle our hips and arms . . .

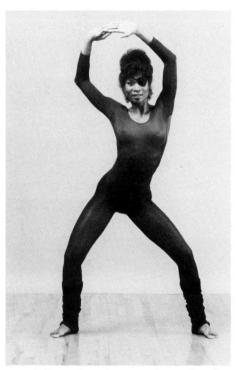

. . . 8 times to relax your lower back.

Repeat all four movements to the left 8 counts in each position, ending with the hip and arm circles.

Breathing: Exhale as you reach out. Inhale as you release between reaches.

Three

WAIST TWISTS
Intercostals, obliques

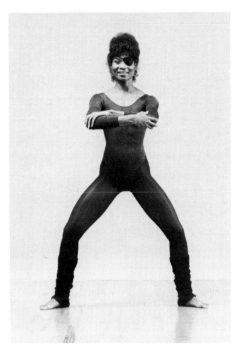

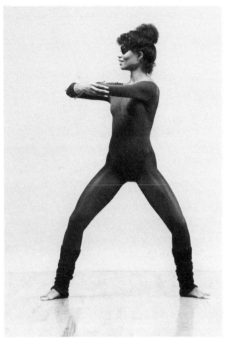

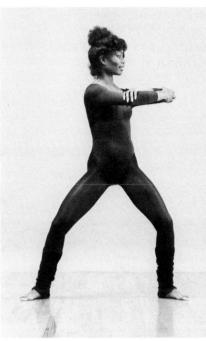

1. Keeping your knees bent . . .

. . . grab your elbows and twist to the right 4 times, releasing slightly between the twists, and looking over your right shoulder.

2. Twist to the left for 4 counts.

Repeat 4 counts to each side.

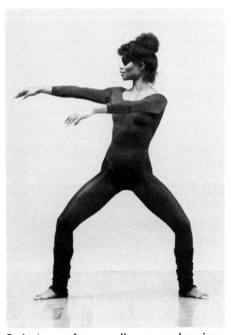

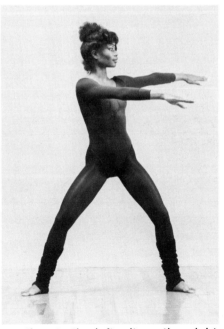

Keep your arms at shoulder heigh during these swings.

Breathing: Steady breathing

3. Let go of your elbows and swing your open arms to the right . . .

. . . then to the left, alternating right and left for a total of 8 swings.

Waist exercises continue on the floor.
Get a mat, towel, blanket—whatever you need to have a soft padding
work out on.

Four
WAIST AND INNER THIGH STRETCH
Intercostals, obliques

Starting position: Sitting on the floor, open your legs as wide as you can without straining the tendons along your inner thighs. Point your toes.

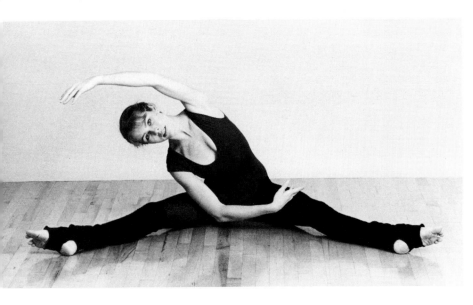

1. Pull over to the right side trying to aim your ear to your leg. Your left arm is pulling directly over to the right while your right arm is gracefully curved in front of you. Bounce gently down, releasing slightly between the bounces, for 8 counts.

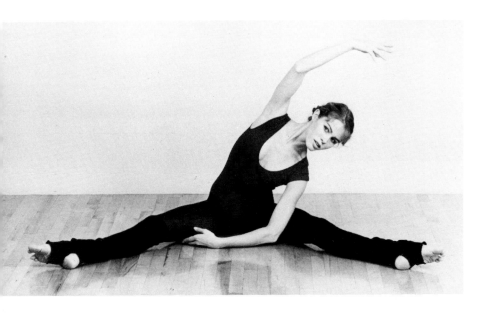

2. Repeat this movement to the left side, bouncing down for 8 counts.

Repeat, alternating sides for 6 counts, then for 4 counts, then repeat twice for 2 counts.

When you are pulling to one side, try to keep the opposite hip on the floor. Be sure to go straight to the side.

Breathing: Exhale as you reach; inhale as you release before reaching.

Five

CHEST-TO-KNEE STRETCH
Intercostals, obliques

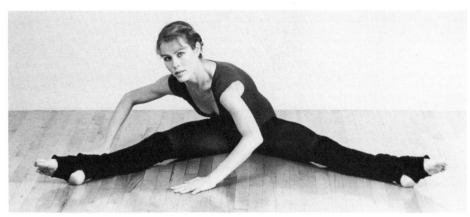

1. Place your hands on each side of your right leg and stretch down reaching the front of your chest toward your knee. Bounce gently for counts.

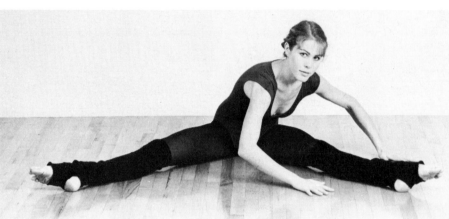

2. With your hands on the floor in front of you, stretch forward out of your hip and "walk" yourself around to the left side. Keep your torso as low as possible to the floor. Take counts to get to the left side. Place your hands on each side of your left leg and stretch down, reaching your chest toward your knee. Bounce gently for 8 counts.

Repeat once to each side.

3. "Walk" to the center again and gently bounce down as low as you can with your hands on the floor in front of you for support and your toes pointed. Bounce for 8 counts.

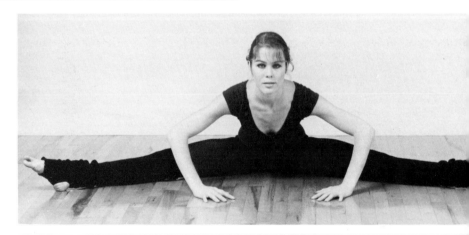

4. Try to open your legs a little wider, flex your feet and bounce gently for another 8 counts.

Breathing: Steady breathing

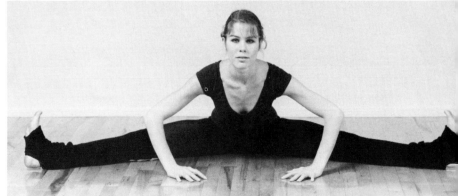

Six

THE KILLER STRETCH
Hamstrings

Starting position: Sitting on the floor, bring your legs together and sit up straight. Grab your toes if you can, your ankles or calves if you can't, and flex your feet so hard your heels are lifted off the floor.

Pull your torso down over your legs as far as you can go. If this stretch is too difficult at first, do it with slightly bent knees.

Hold for 10 counts.

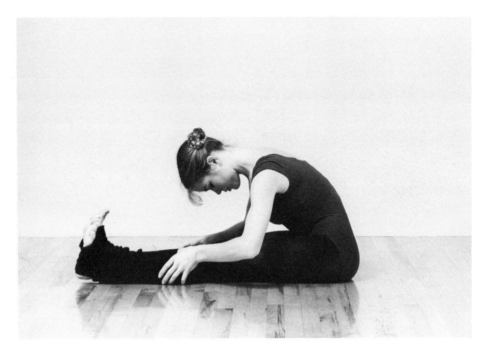

Breathing: Inhale deeply to begin, then exhale deeply as you pull down, to relax and lengthen the stretch.

Shake your legs out by slapping them against the floor a few times.

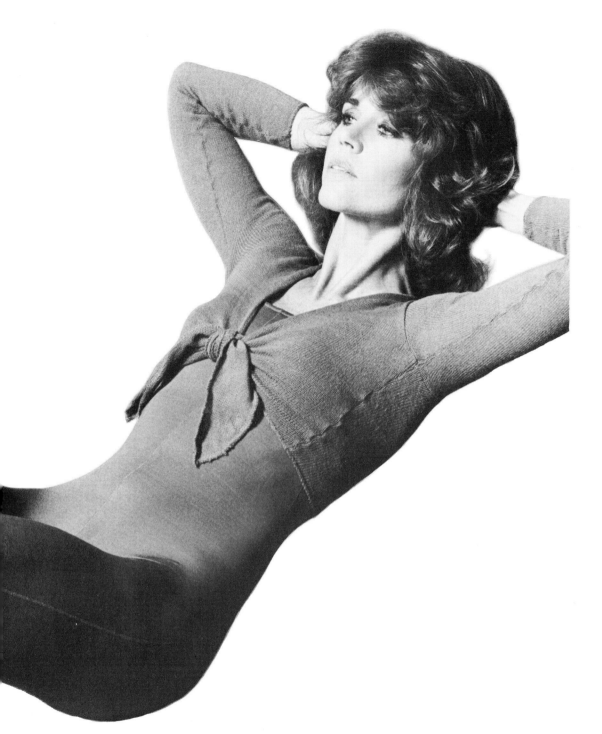

Beginners'
ABDOMINALS

ABDOMINALS 4 MINUTES

Purpose:
To burn away the spare tire, tone and strengthen the upper and lower abdominal muscles.

Music:
Linda Clifford—"Bridge Over Troubled Water"/*Let Me Be Your Woman*
Blondie—"Call Me"/*American Gigolo*
Irene Cara—"Fame"/*Fame*
Irene Cara—"Red Light"/*Fame*
Sylvester—"You Make Me Feel"/*Step 2*
Sylvester—"Dance Disco Heat"/*Step 2*
Voyage—"Souvenirs"/*Night at Studio 54*
Musique—"In the Bush"/*Night at Studio 54*
D. C. LaRue—"Hot Jungle Drums & Voodoo Rhythm"/*Night at Studio 54*
Evelyn "Champagne" King—"Shame"/*Smooth Talk*
Evelyn "Champagne" King—"Nobody Knows"/*Smooth Talk*
Gloria Gaynor—"I Will Survive"/*Love Tracks*

Note of caution: You must concentrate on keeping your stomach pulled in during all these exercises, so as not to develop a protruding abdomen.

One

SIT-UPS
Lower abdominals

Starting position: Lie on your back, knees bent, feet flat on floor, feet and knees parallel about a foot apart, hands behind your head with your elbows out to the sides.

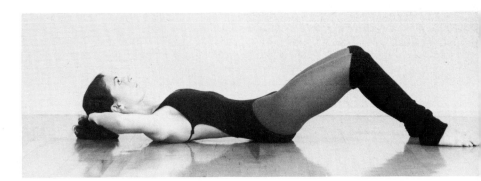

1. Lift your head and upper back off the floor as high as you can, using your abdominal muscles, not your arms. Keep your elbows back.

2. Lower a little but do not touch the floor.

Do these lifts, combining movements 1 and 2, 20 times.

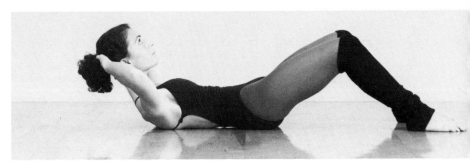

Breathing: Exhale as you lift, inhale as you lower.

Two

THROUGH LEG REACHES
Upper and lower abdominals

Leave your right hand behind your head for support and reach through your knees with the left arm, pulling through, releasing slightly between pulls, for 15 counts.

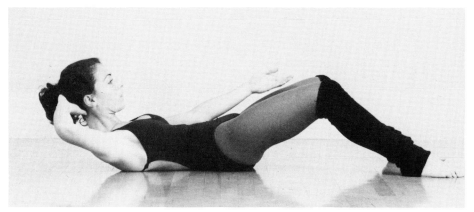

Breathing: Exhale as you reach; inhale as you release slightly between reaches.

Three

KNEES TO CHEST
Abdominal release

Starting position: Continuing from preceding exercise, let the head relax back onto the floor.

Hug your knees tightly in to your chest and hold for 10 counts. This position is especially soothing and beneficial for the female organs.

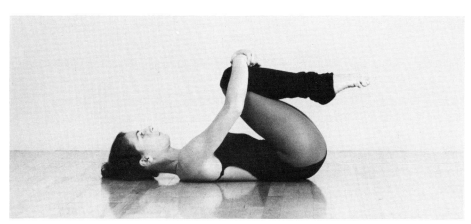

Breathing: Normal

Four

THE BICYCLE
Obliques, lower abdominals

1. Place your hands behind your head and extend the right leg straight out, a few inches off the floor, toes pointed. Bend your left knee in to your chest, reaching your right elbow to touch your left knee.

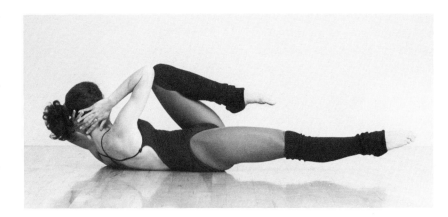

2. Switch sides, extending the left leg out with toe pointed. Bend the right knee in and touch the left elbow to the right knee.

These two movements, right and left, are done to one count. Repeat for a total of 10 counts with toes pointed,

... then do 10 times with feet flexed.

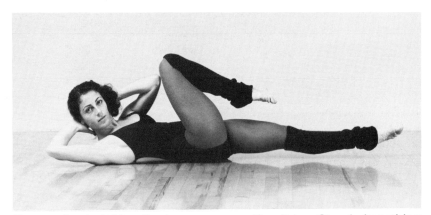

Be sure to straighten the leg as you extend it, and keep it close to the floor.

Breathing: Steady breathing

Five

KNEES TO CHEST
Abdominal release

Starting position: Let the head and upper body relax back onto the floor.

Hug your knees tightly in to your chest, holding for 10 counts.

Breathing: Normal

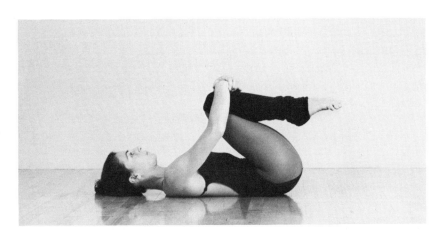

Six

EXTENDED LEG SIT-UPS
Lower and upper abdominals

Starting position: Extend your legs toward the ceiling with knees slightly bent, hands behind your head with your elbows back.

1. Lift your head and upper torso using your abdominal muscles, not your arms.

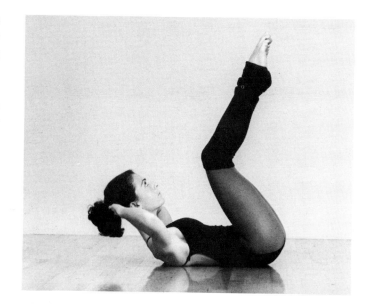

2. Then release back slightly but don't let your head or shoulders touch the floor.

Do these two movements 20 times.

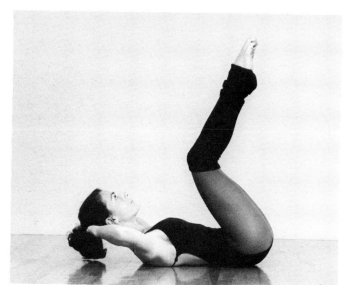

3. Lift up even farther, extending your arms past your lifted legs. Keep your knees slightly bent. Lift like this—reach, release, reach, release—for 30 counts.

Breathing: Exhale as you reach. Inhale as you release slightly between reaches.

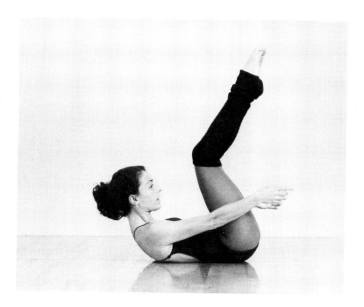

Seven KNEES TO CHEST
Abdominal release

Starting position: Let the head and upper body relax back onto the floor.

Hug your knees tightly in to your chest, holding for 10 counts.

Breathing: Normal

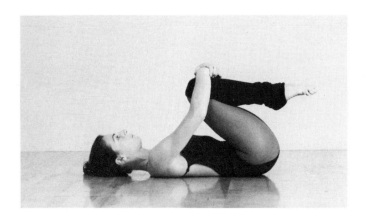

Eight EXTENDED SCISSOR KICKS
Upper and lower abdominals, quadriceps

Starting position: Extend your legs straight up in the air with toes pointed and place your hands behind your head, elbows back.

1. Lift your head up as far as possible and cross your right leg over the left leg.

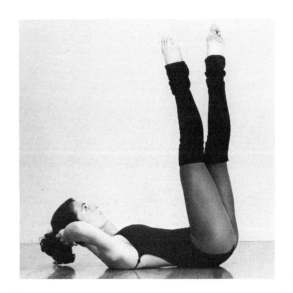

2. Then cross the left leg over the right in a rapid scissoring motion.

These two movements are done to one count. Scissor for 10 counts with toes pointed,

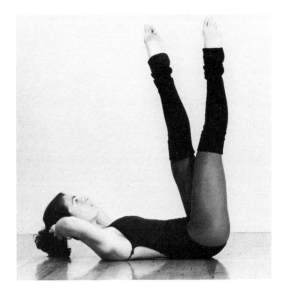

3. . . . then 10 counts with toes flexed.

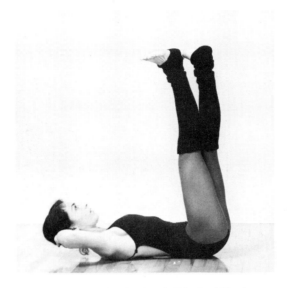

Keep your head off the floor. Use your abdominal muscles to hold your head up; don't rely on your arms.

Breathing: Steady breathing

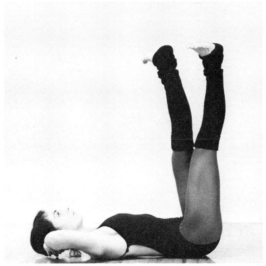

Nine   KNEES TO CHEST
Abdominal release

Starting position: Let the head and upper body relax back onto the floor.

Hug your knees tightly in to your chest for 10 counts.

Breathing: Normal

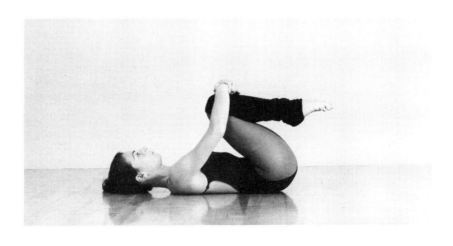

Ten

STOMACH RELEASE
To release abdominals and lower back

1. Swing your knees over to the right side and your arms to the left.

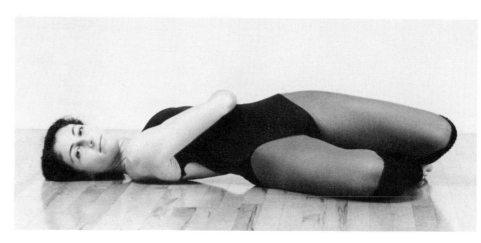

2. Swing your knees over to the left side and your arms to the right.

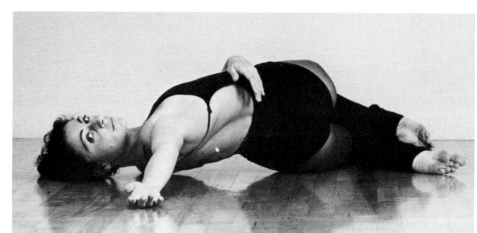

Repeat once to each side.

Breathing: Normal

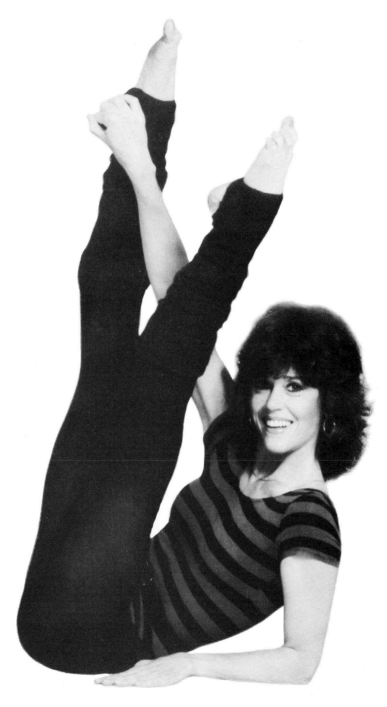

Beginners'
LEGS AND HIPS

LEGS AND HIPS 4 MINUTES

Purpose:
To burn off the fatty deposits, tone and strengthen the muscles on the sides o
the hips and thighs, the troublesome inner thighs, and the back of the hips. These
are the best, most effective exercises I've ever found for these problem areas

Music:
Dolly Parton—"Baby I'm Burnin' "/*Heartbreaker*
Fleetwood Mac—"Dreams"/*Rumours*
Brothers Johnson—"Stomp"/*Light Up the Night*
Eddie Rabbitt—"I Love a Rainy Night"/*Horizon*
Chic—"Le Freak"/*C'est Chic*
Taste of Honey—"Boogie Oogie Oogie"/*Taste of Honey*
Jacksons—"Shake Your Body Down"/*Destiny*
Paul Jabara—"Shut Out"/*Perils of Paul*
Linda Clifford—"One of Those Songs"/*Let Me Be Your Woman*

One

LEG LIFTS TO THE SIDE
Gluteus medius, gluteus minimus, tensor fasciae latae

Starting position: Lie on your left side, up on your left elbow, palms flat on the floor. Extend both legs straight out on a line with your upper body.

1. With toes pointed, lift your right leg up.

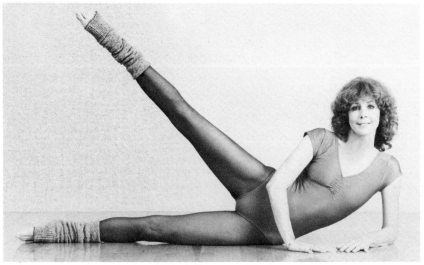

MODEL—SHIRLEE FONDA

2. Lower your right leg but don't let it touch your bottom leg.

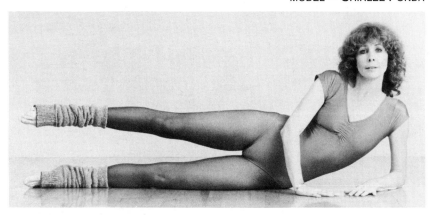

116

Do this 15 times with your toes pointed.

Repeat 15 times with your toes flexed.

Breathing: Exhale as leg lifts up, inhale as leg lowers.

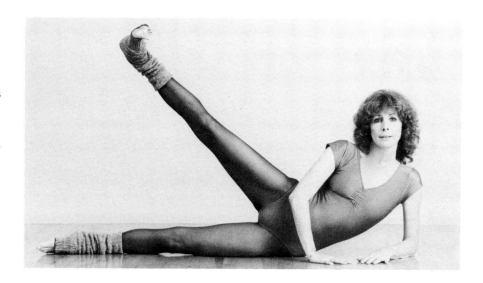

Two

KNEE IN, LEG UP
Gluteus medius, gluteus minimus, tensor fasciae latae

1. Bend your right knee in to your body.

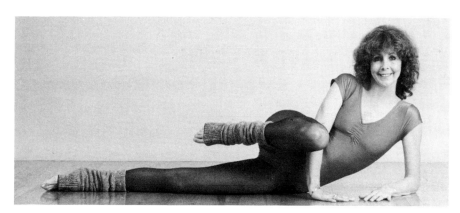

2. Extend your right leg straight out again, on a line with your left leg.

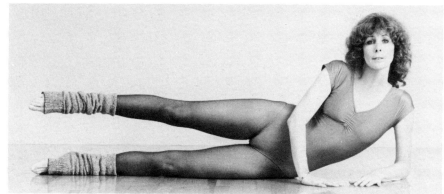

3. Lift your right leg straight up.

These three movements are done to one count. Repeat for a total of 5 counts.

Breathing: Exhale as leg extends, inhale as knee bends in.

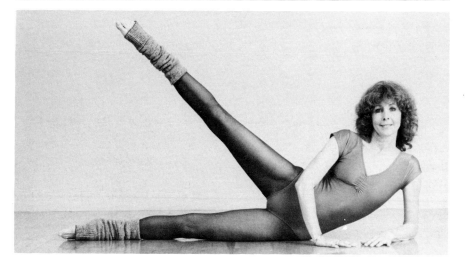

Three

CROSSOVERS

Gluteus maximus, medius, minimus, tensor fasciae latae and quadriceps

1. Bend your bottom leg, trying to align your thigh with your upper body. Grab your right knee with your right hand and pull your knee in to your chest.

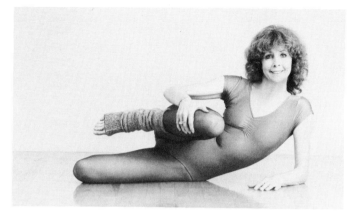

2. Extend your right leg out from your body at a slight angle. Turn your toes down so that your heel is higher than your toes.

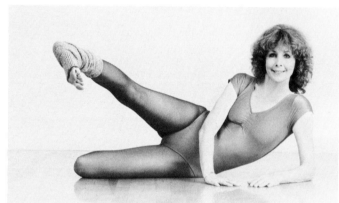

3. Lower your right leg to within a few inches of the floor.

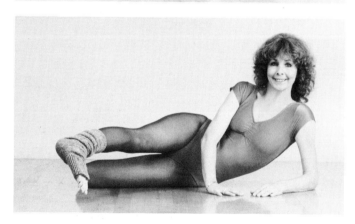

4. Raise your right leg up again.

Do this exercise 15 times slowly and 15 times double-time.

Be sure to move the leg from the hip. Don't let the knee bend and, *most emphatically*, do not move the rest of the body. This is not an easy exercise and as you begin to tire there will be a tendency to raise and lower your leg by throwing your hips into it. Try feeling there's a wall against your back and you cannot rock your hips back.

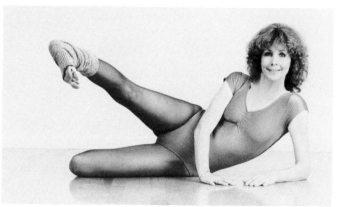

Go for the burn! You'll like the results.

Breathing: Exhale as leg lowers, inhale as leg raises.

Four

BACK LEG LIFTS
Gluteus maximus, hamstrings

Starting position: Roll over so that your hips and chest are facing the floor. Come up on your left elbow and reach your right arm out in front of you. Extend both legs, knees straight, toes pointed. Cross the right leg over the left.

Lift your right leg as high as you can with toe pointed. Release it a little but don't let it drop too low. This is a small movement: lifting your leg from a lifted position. It will also strengthen your back.

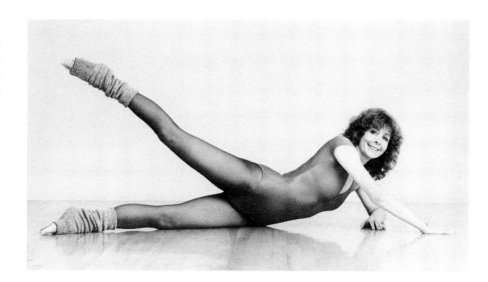

Do 10 counts with toes pointed and 10 counts with foot flexed.

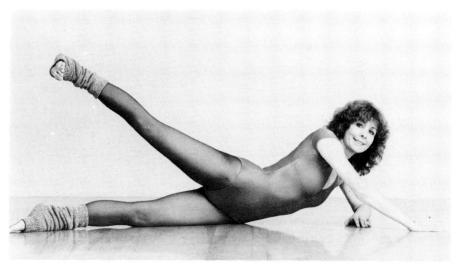

Breathing: Exhale as leg lifts, inhale as it releases.

Five

QUAD STRETCH
Stretches quadriceps

1. After the final back leg lift, reach around with your right hand and grab your right foot, stretching it in to your buttocks.

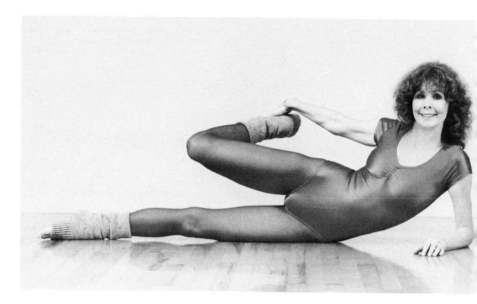

2. Then roll over onto your back, come up on your elbows, palms of your hands flat on the floor with your right leg bent under you. Stay in this position 8 counts pushing your right knee down and your right hip up. Feel the stretch up the front of your thigh.

Breathing: Normal

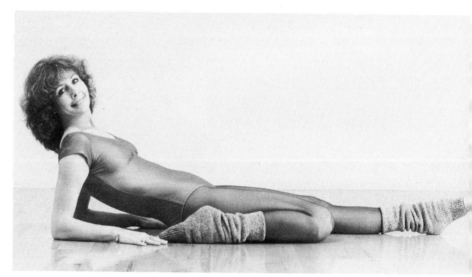

Six

INNER THIGH LIFTS
Adductor magnus, adductor brevis, adductor longus, gracilis, pectineus

Starting position: Come back up onto your left side. Bend your left elbow. Grab your right foot with your right hand and bring it in front of your left leg which is extended an inch off the floor with toes pointed.

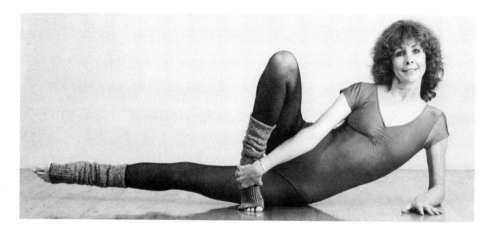

1. Lift your left leg, lowering it slightly between lifts, for 10 counts with toes pointed.

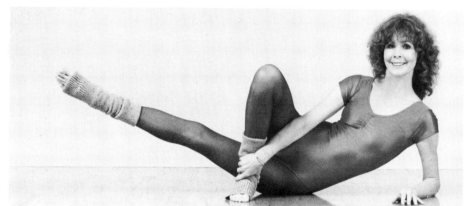

2. Repeat, same leg, for 10 counts with foot flexed.

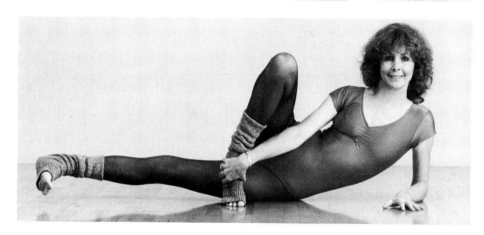

Be sure your left leg is turned out so that the inner thigh is facing the ceiling.

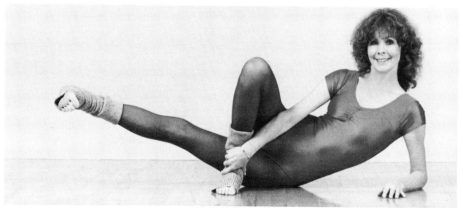

Breathing: Exhale as leg lifts, inhale as it lowers between lifts.

Seven

HIP RELEASE
Gluteus maximus

Starting position: Sit cross-legged on the floor, right foot in front of the left foot.

Round down over your bent legs and hold for 10 counts, then roll back up.

Breathing: Normal

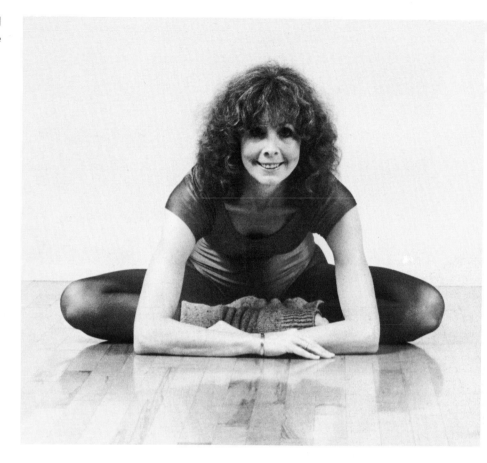

Now you will repeat the entire sequence of leg and hip exercises (Exercises One through Seven) to the other side.

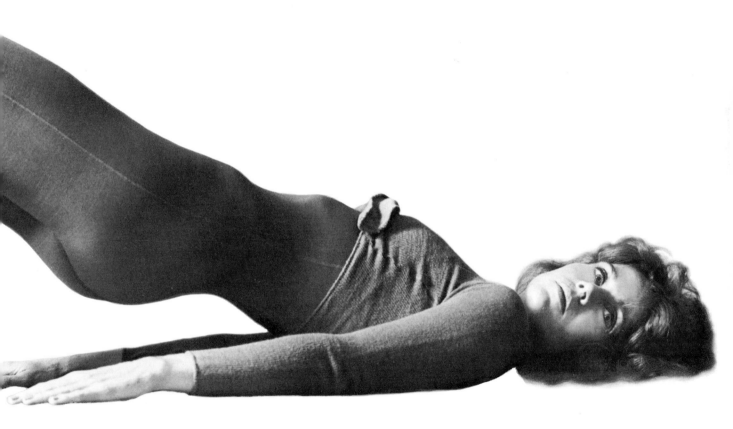

Beginners'
BUTTOCKS

BUTTOCKS 2 MINUTES

Purpose: To trim, tone and firm the buttocks (gluteus maximus, medius and minimus, biceps femoris). If you're eating properly, these exercises will give you a smaller, firmer butt, less apt to "fall," and those saddlebags will disappear.

Music:
Bob Seger—"Against the Wind"/*Against the Wind*
Sister Sledge—"We Are Family"/*We Are Family*
Michael Jackson—"Rock With You"/*Off the Wall*
Santana—"Stormy"/*Inner Secrets*
Cheryl Lynn—"Got to Be Real"/*Night at Studio 54*
Pointer Sisters—"Hypnotized"/*Energy*
Olivia Newton-John—"Totally Hot"/*Totally Hot*
Ralph McDonald—"Calypso"/*Saturday Night Fever*

One BUTTOCKS LIFTS

Starting position: Lie on your back, feet parallel, a little more than hip distance apart, your arms lying alongside your body.

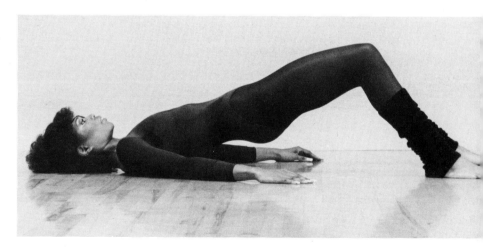

1. With knees and feet parallel, shift your weight onto your shoulders and lift your buttocks up . . .

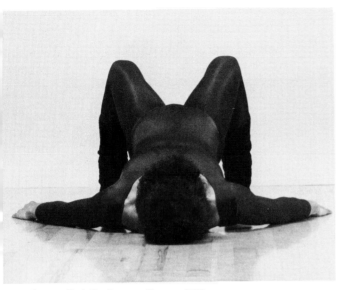

. . . then slightly lower them, lifting and lowering for 10 counts.

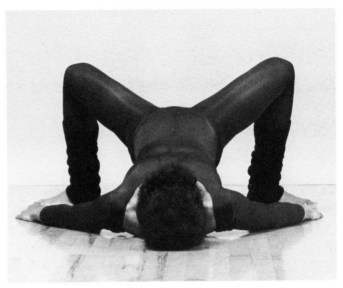

2. Turn your knees and feet out (let them drop open) and continue lifting and slightly lowering your buttocks for 10 counts.

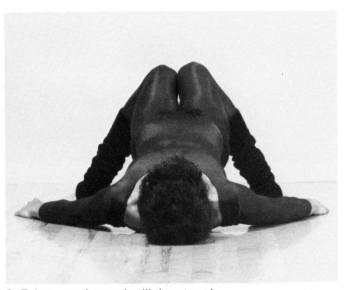

3. Bring your knees in till they touch, as you push up hard with your buttocks. (Resist bringing your knees in. Make it hard so you'll really work your outer and inner thighs as well as your buttocks. You should feel the burn all the way down the inner thigh to the knee.)

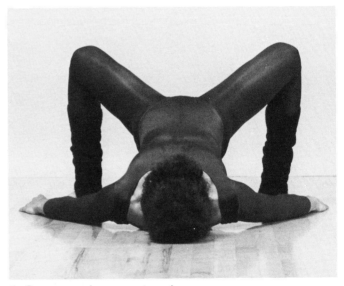

4. Open your knees out again as you slightly relax your buttocks muscles.

These two movements, 3 and 4, are done to one count. Repeat for a total of 10 counts.

Breathing: For movements 3 and 4, exhale as knees come together, inhale as knees open.

CONTINUED→

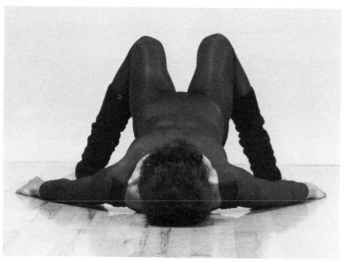

5. Rapidly bounce your knees together for 10 counts.

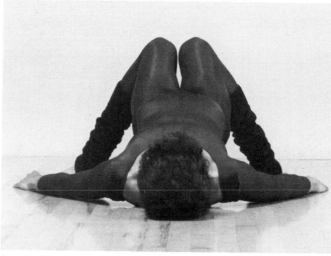

As you bounce the knees together keep pushing up as hard as you can with your buttocks. Go for the burn! I know it hurts but you'll feel so good afterwards, and you'll be so pleased with the results.

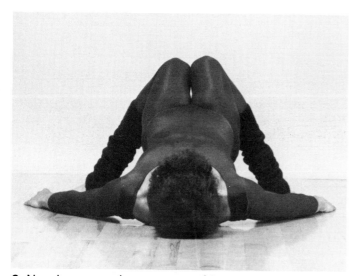

6. Now keep your knees pressed together as you continue to lift and lower your buttocks for 10 counts. Work deep!

Breathing: Exhale as you lift; inhale as you lower between the lifts.

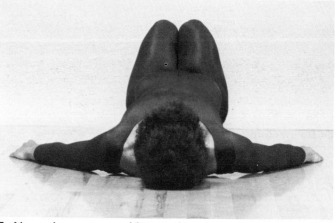

7. Now place your ankles and your knees together and lift for a final 10 counts. Whew!

This lifting movement should be very small. What counts is the intensity. You have to work deep. If it burns too much, stop for a brief moment and start again. If your back aches during this series, it means you are arching it. In this case concentrate on rounding your lower back as you lift your buttocks.

Two   HIP RELEASE AND STRETCH
Hamstrings, gluteus maximus

Starting position: Lower hips to floor.

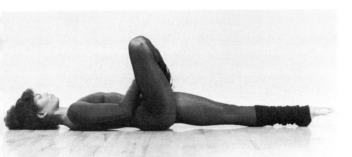

1. Extend your left leg out on the floor with the toe pointed. Grab your right foot with both hands and pull the foot across your body, stretching your right hip. This should feel good after what you've just done. Pull gently for 4 counts.

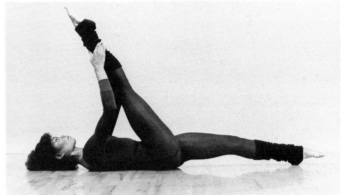

2. Extend your right leg up toward your head with a straight knee and pull it toward you with both hands for 4 counts.

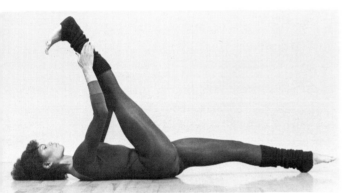

3. Point and flex your foot twice as you pull your leg in to your body.

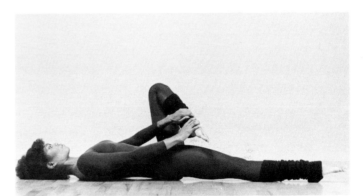

4. Change legs, extending your right leg out on the floor while grabbing your left foot with both hands and pulling it across your body for 4 counts.

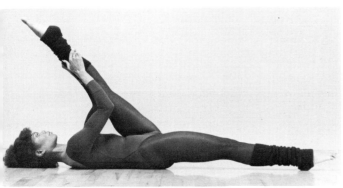

5. Extend your left leg up toward your head and pull it toward you with both hands for 4 counts.

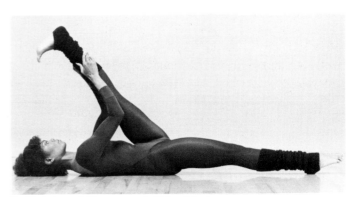

6. Point and flex your left foot twice as you pull your leg to your body.

Breathing: Normal

Three   HIP AND THIGH RELEASE
Inner thigh

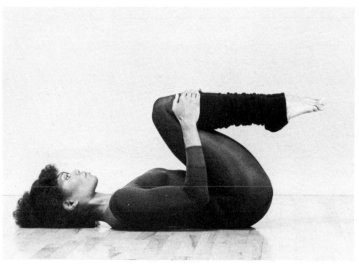

1. Bend both knees in to your torso, pulling them in with your hands.

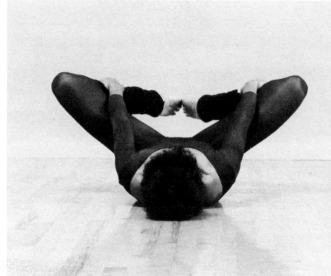

2. Open your knees out to the side, grab both lower legs and press down gently, releasing slightly between presses, for 8 counts.

3. Open your legs wide out to the sides, hold on to your ankles or calves and gently bounce down for 16 counts.

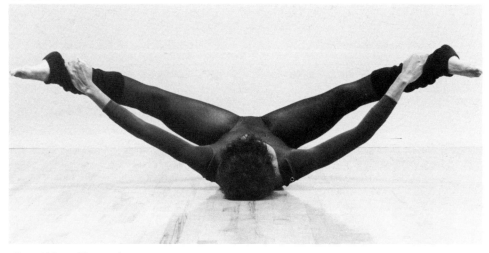

Breathing: Normal

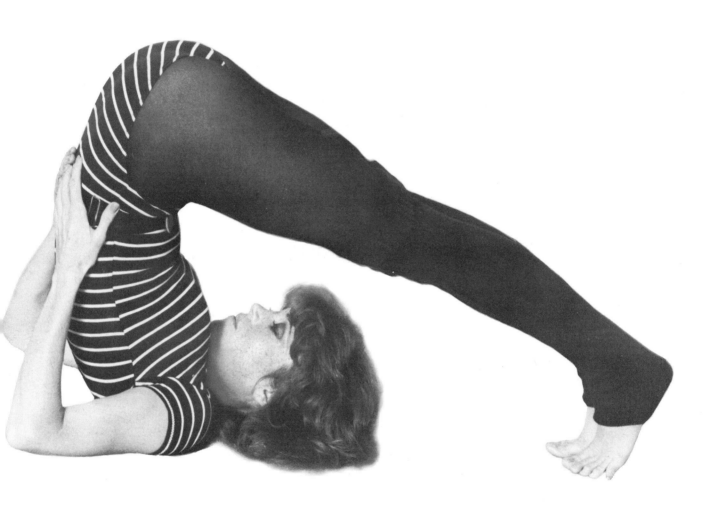

Beginners'
COOL-DOWN

COOL-DOWN 3 MINUTES

Purpose: To allow your pulse rate to return to normal and to finish your workout with some excellent yoga stretches.

Music:
Karla Bonoff—"Falling Star"/*Bonoff, Karla*
Karla Bonoff—"Roses in the Garden"/*Bonoff, Karla*
Boz Scaggs—"Harbor Lights"/*Silk Degrees*
Judy Collins—"Houses"/*Judith*
Dan Fogelberg—"Souvenirs"/*Souvenirs*
Jean-François Paillard Chamber Orchestra—"Canon in D"/*Pachelbel—Canon in D*

One THE FROG

Starting position: Lie on your back, bend your knees outward, press the soles of your feet together and lower your thighs to the floor.

Relax the inner thighs and press the small of the back into the floor.

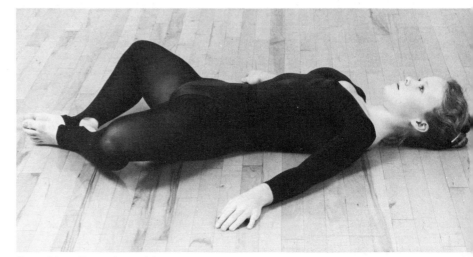

Breathing: Deep breathing

Two

THE PLOUGH

1. Pull your knees in to your chest.

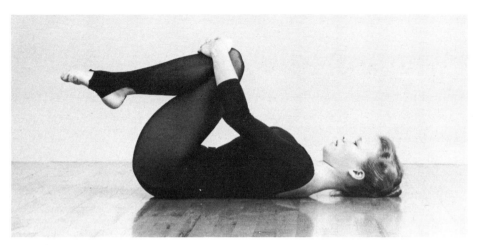

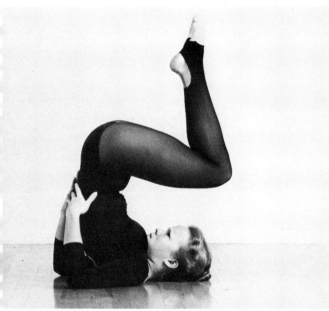

2. Lift your hips up, supporting your lower back with your hands. Bend your knees over your head.

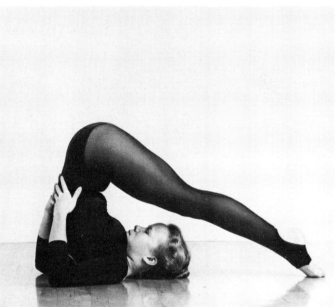

3. Extend your straight legs out past your head as far as you can with pointed toes, feet touching the floor behind your head. Support your lower back with your hands. Hold this position a minute or two if you can.

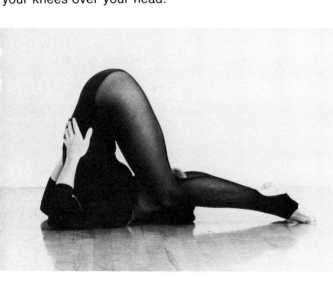

4. Drop your knees next to your ears and hold for a minute.

CONTINUED→

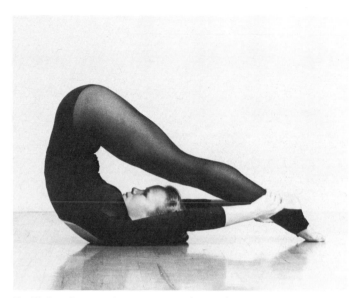

5. Extend your legs out again and grab your ankles with both hands.

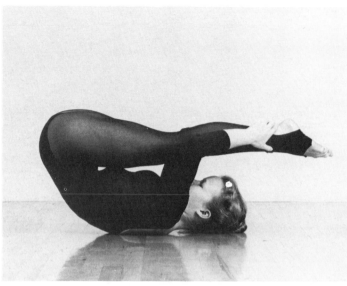

6. Begin to roll down one vertebra at a time. Control your speed by holding your ankles and dragging your legs across your face.

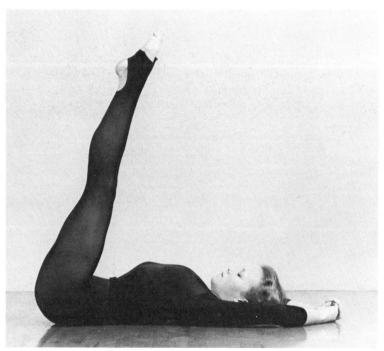

7. When the small of your back is on the floor, let go of your legs.

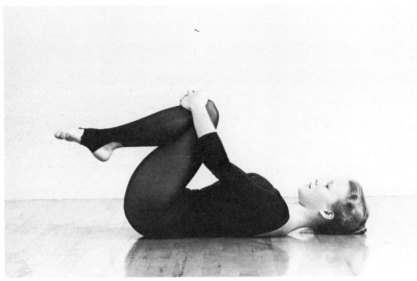

8. Grab your knees and hug them tightly to your chest.

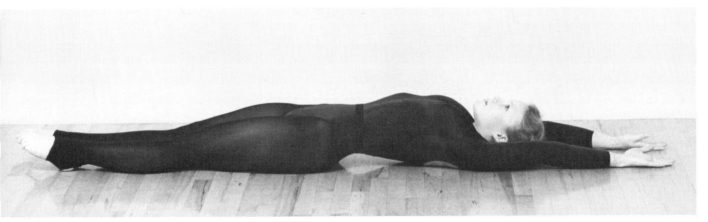

9. Extend your legs and arms and stretch out as far as you can, legs in one direction, arms in the other.

Breathing: Normal

The yoga Plough position is one of the best stretches you can do. It stretches out the spine, allows the vital energy flow to be opened up and, because the chin is being pressed into the chest, stimulates the thyroid gland at the base of the neck. This is the gland that regulates your metabolism.

This is a good position to take when you're tired. If you hold it for two minutes and come down very very slowly, you will feel refreshed.

CONCENTRATE ON WHAT YOU ARE DOING

**NO DISTRACTIONS
CENTER YOURSELF
THIS IS *YOUR* TIME**

Perform these exercises to music by The Jacksons,
REO Speedwagon, Brothers Johnson and many more
on my Workout Record and Workout Tape, available on
the CBS label in all good department stores and record
shops in the UK.

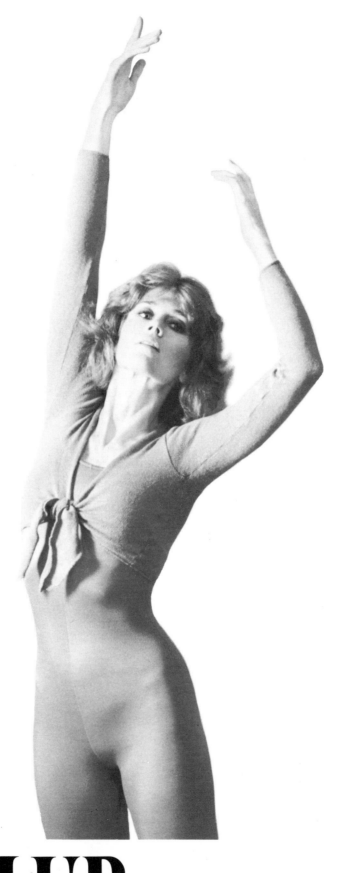

Advanced
WARM-UP

WARM-UP 5 MINUTES

Purpose:
To increase the pulse rate, heat up and stretch out the muscles in every part of the body. No exercise session should begin without warming up. Cold muscles are more easily injured.

Music:
London Symphony Orchestra—"Theme from *Star Wars*"/*Star Wars*
Donna Summer—"Fairy Tale High"/*Live and More*
Irene Cara—"Red Light"/*Fame*
Kongas—"Gimme Some Lovin' "/*Africanism*
Barbra Streisand—"Main Event"/*Main Event*

One HEAD ROLLS

Starting position: Standing erect, place feet a little more than hip distance apart. Pull up out of the hips, stomach pulled in, buttocks squeezed tight, shoulders down, arms at sides.

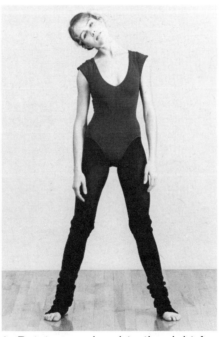

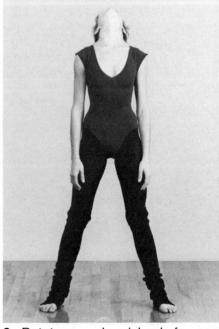

1. Rotate your head to the right for one count. Feel the stretch up the left side of your neck. Don't let your shoulders hunch up.

2. Rotate your head back for one count. Stretch your chin to the ceiling and let your mouth open.

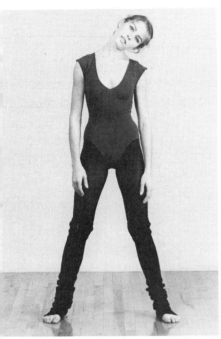 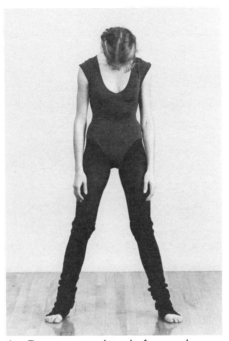

Repeat the same movement to the right again taking one count for each position, then reverse and do the same thing two times to the left.

Breathing: Normal

3. Rotate your head to the left one count.

4. Drop your head forward one count, stretching your chin to your chest. Feel the pull up the back of your neck.

Two SHOULDER LIFTS

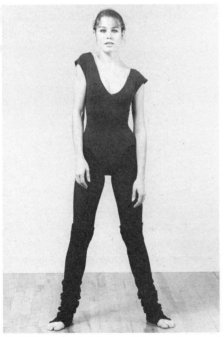 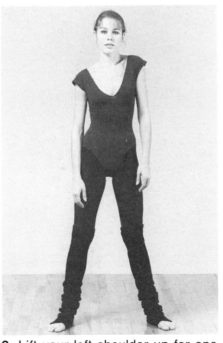

Repeat right and left shoulder lifts for a total of 8 counts.

Breathing: Normal

1. Lift your right shoulder up toward your ear for one count.

2. Lift your left shoulder up for one count as you lower your right shoulder.

Three SIDE STRETCHES

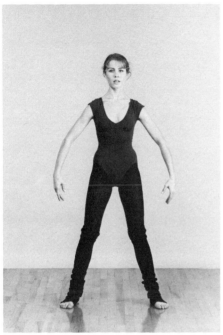

1. Inhale as you open your arms to the side.

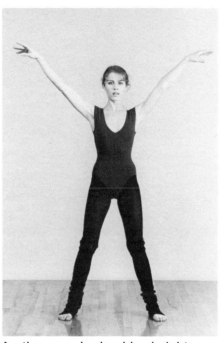

As they reach shoulder height, exhale . . .

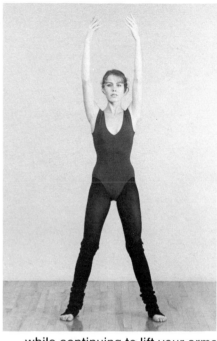

. . . while continuing to lift your arms over your head.

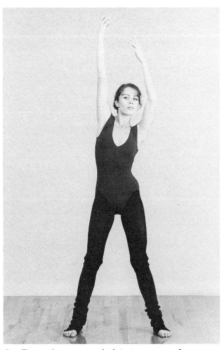

2. Reach your right arm as far upward toward the ceiling as you can for one count. Feel the stretch up your right side.

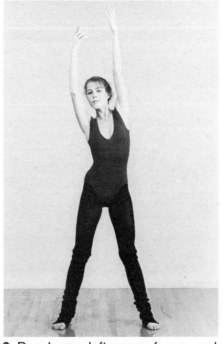

3. Reach your left arm as far upward as you can for one count. Feel the stretch up your left side.

Repeat, reaching right and left for a total of 8 counts.

Breathing: Exhale as you reach, inhale as you change arms.

Four

WAIST REACHES

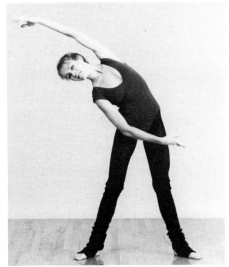

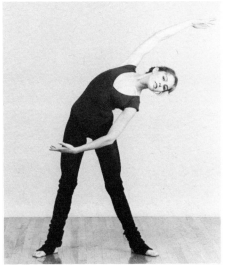

1. Pulling outward and directly to the side, reach your left arm over your head to the right. Gently bounce for 4 counts, keeping hips forward, left shoulder back, and right arm curved in front of you.

2. Reach your right arm over your head to the left and bounce for 4 counts, curving your left arm in front of you.

Repeat once to the right and once to the left.

Breathing: Normal

Five

HAMSTRING STRETCHES

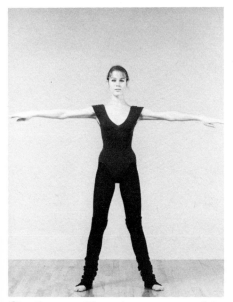

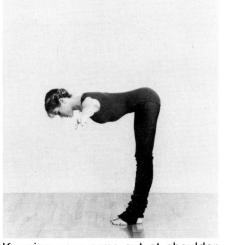

Starting position: As you complete the final reach to the left in the preceding exercise, come back to center position, opening your arms to shoulder height for 2 counts while you inhale.

Keeping your arms out at shoulder height, take 4 counts to bend forward with a flat back and straight legs. Exhale as you bend forward. Stretch your chin outward, your buttocks to the ceiling and "pulse" the small of your back downward in little bounces for a count of 8.

Breathing: Normal

Six HAMSTRING STRETCHES

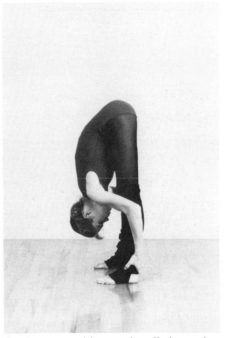

Breathing: Normal. Careful, don't hold your breath.

Grab your ankles and pull down for 8 counts.

Seven SPINE STRETCH

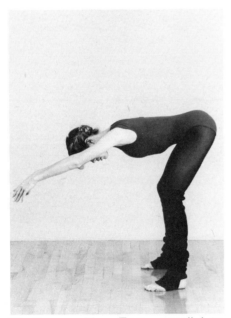

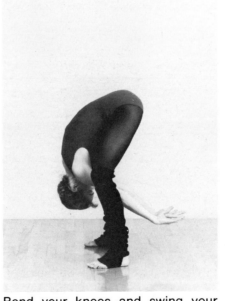

Breathing: Exhale as you swing through legs, inhale as you come up to starting position.

Starting position: Torso parallel to floor, arms stretched, knees bent.

Bend your knees and swing your arms through your legs and return to starting position 8 times. Take one count for each swing through and return.

Eight

HAMSTRING STRETCHES

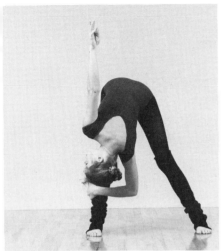

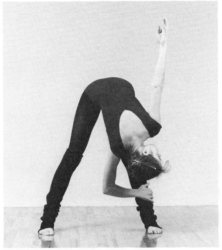

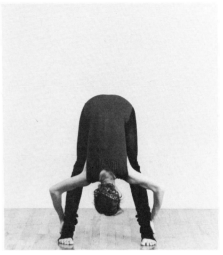

1. Straighten your legs again and grab your right ankle with your left hand and pull your torso down over your right leg. Let your right arm reach up toward the ceiling. Pull down this way, thinking of stretching your chest to your knee, for 4 counts.

2. Repeat the same movement to the left side for 4 counts, grabbing your left ankle with your right hand and letting your left arm reach upward.

Repeat 4 counts right, 4 counts left.

3. Come center, grab both ankles and pull down 4 counts.

Breathing: Steady breathing

Nine

HAMSTRING STRETCHES

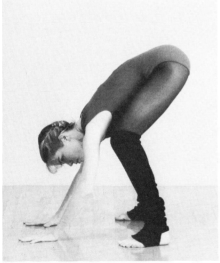

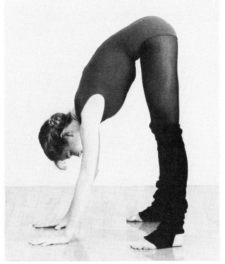

Starting position: Bend your knees, feet apart, and place your hands on the floor in front of you.

Straighten and bend your knees trying to keep your hands on the floor. The two movements—bending and straightening—are done to one count. Do this for 8 counts.

Breathing: Exhale as you straighten, inhale as you bend.

Ten CALF RAISES

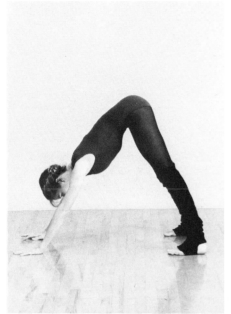 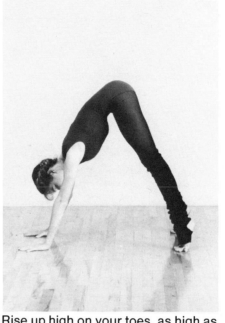

Starting position: Keep your feet apart, walk your hands away from your body, and keep your knees straight.

Rise up high on your toes, as high as you possibly can to really work your ankles and calves, then lower your heels again.

Do this 30 times. Go for the burn!

Breathing: Exhale as you rise on your toes, inhale as you lower heels.

Eleven INNER THIGH STRETCH

Starting position: Walk your hands back in between your legs, bend your knees into a squatting position and place your hands behind your feet. You'll find your inner knees are resting on your elbows, which should stretch your inner thighs open.

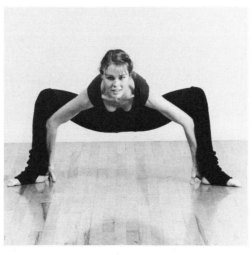

Small bounces with your buttocks for 16 counts.

Breathing: Normal

Twelve ROLL-UP

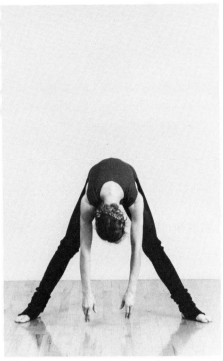

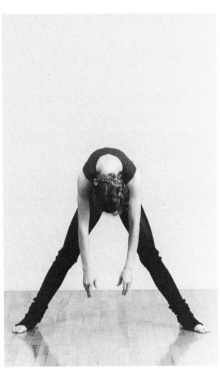

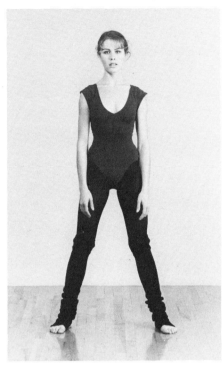

Starting position: Let go of your feet, straighten your knees, let your arms and head hang limp like a rag doll.

Slowly roll up, one vertebra at a time,

. . . until you are standing straight and erect, exactly as you began the warm-up.

Breathing: Normal

Thirteen AEROBIC SERIES

Purpose:

This aerobic section is part of the warm-up. Now that you have begun to limber up and get the blood flowing, you will further increase your pulse rate, burn up some calories and begin to strengthen your heart and lungs. It will be difficult at first, but hang in there. Before long, it will seem easy and as you build cardio-vascular strength you will feel tremendous exhilaration and increased energy.

It is crucial that you remember to breathe deeply and regularly all during these exercises. As the heart is called upon to pump blood faster to your muscles, your lungs must send larger amounts of oxygen into the bloodstream to be carried to the muscles and to carry away the waste gases.

Music:

Continue with the same music used in the beginning of the warm-up.

Starting position: Standing erect, feet together, pull up out of the torso.

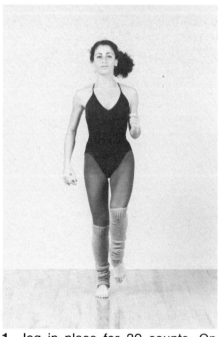

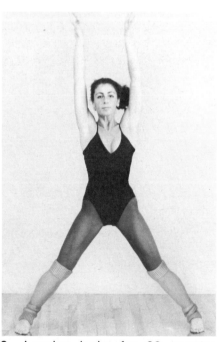

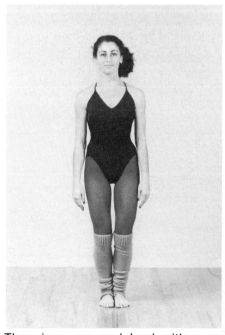

1. Jog in place for 20 counts. On each count both the right and left feet touch down. You should land on the balls of your feet and then work through the whole foot, being sure to let the heels touch down.

2. Jumping jacks for 20 counts: Jump up and open your legs, landing with your legs apart as your arms swing out to the side and up over your head.

Then jump up and land with your feet together as you bring your arms down to your sides again. These two jumps are done to one count.

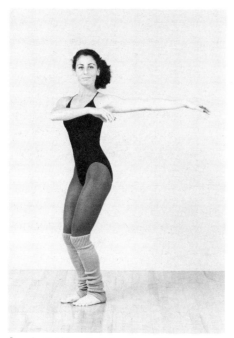

3. Jumping twists for 10 counts: Jump and twist your body to the right as you swing your arms to the left,

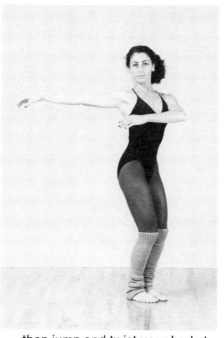

. . . then jump and twist your body to the left swinging your arms to the right. These two movements are done to one count.

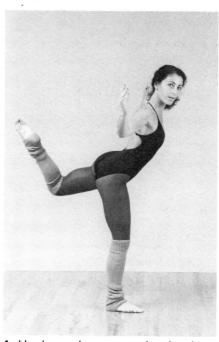

4. Heels up, knees up: Jog in place for 5 counts, lifting your heels up behind you.

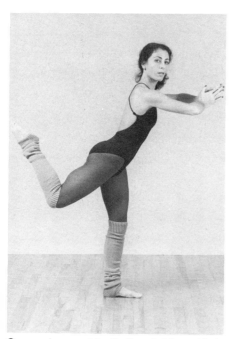

On each count both the right and left heels lift up.

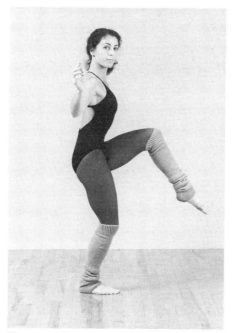

Then, while you continue jogging in place, prance for 5 counts, lifting your knees high in front of you.

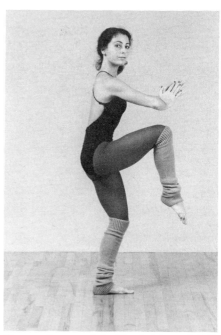

On each count both right and left knees lift. Repeat 5 counts heels up, 5 counts knees up. Clap your hands when the right leg lifts on each count.

CONTINUED→

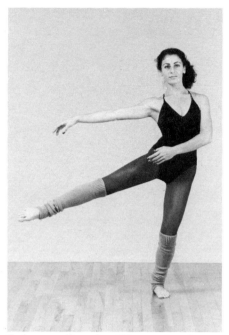

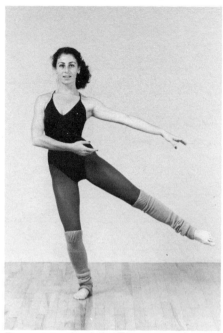

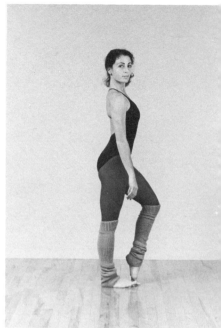

5. Leg swings for 20 counts: Jump, landing on your left foot, and swing your right leg and your arms out to the right side.

Repeat to the left. These two jumps are done to one count.

6. Jog in place again for 20 counts, slowing down until only your heels are lifting off the floor, to allow the pulse rate to gradually slow down.

Fourteen   ROLL-DOWN AND KNEE BENDS

Starting position: Feet together, arms hanging at your sides, stomach pulled in, buttocks tight.

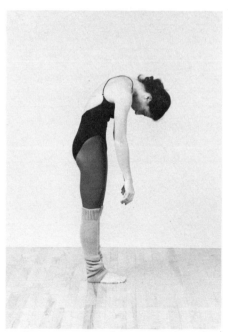

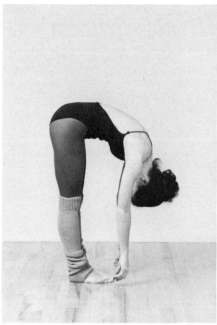

1. Drop your head forward, keeping your knees straight, and roll down one vertebra at a time. Let your arms hang limp like a rag doll.

Take 4 counts for hands to touch the floor.

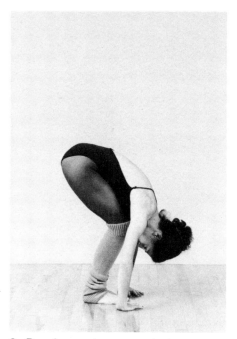

2. Bend your knees and place your hands on the floor.

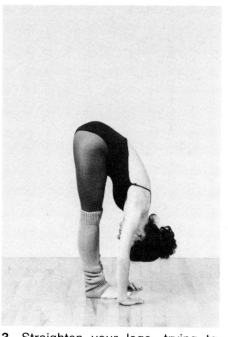

3. Straighten your legs, trying to keep your hands on the floor. Bend and straighten to one count. Do this for 8 counts.

Breathing: Exhale as you straighten your knees. Inhale as you bend them.

Fifteen TENDON STRETCH

Starting position: Walk your hands way out in front of you. Straighten both legs.

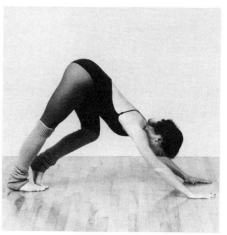

1. Lift your left heel up, bending the left knee, while you bounce your right heel to the floor for 4 counts.

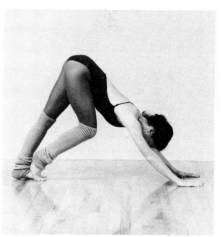

2. Lift your right heel up, bending the right knee and straightening the left, while you bounce your left heel to the floor for 4 counts.

Repeat 3 times to each side, alternating right and left.

Breathing: Normal

Sixteen JAZZ STRETCH

Starting position: Bring your right foot forward in a "lunge" with your left leg stretched out behind you. Try not to bend the back leg. Your hands are on the floor on either side of your front leg.

1. Bounce forward for 4 counts. Feel the stretch in the hip and the front of the back thigh. Be sure the front heel is on the floor.

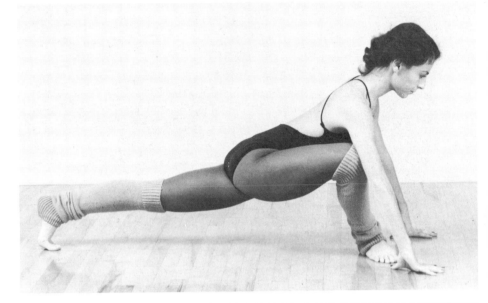

2. Rock back so that your front leg is straight and your front foot is flexed. Pull your chest down to your knee (or try to) for 4 counts.

Repeat the forward and back positions (1 and 2) 3 times.

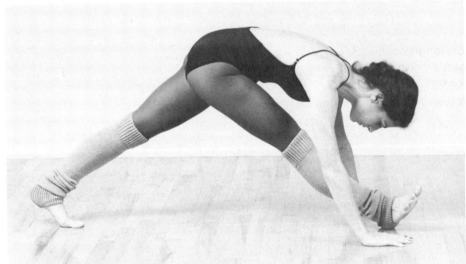

3. As you finish pulling your chest to your front leg for the third time, place the toes of your front foot on the floor and pull down toward your foot even farther. Hold for 8 counts. Keep your back leg straight.

Bring your right foot back, place your left foot forward and repeat the 3 movements to the other side.

Breathing: Take a breath so you can exhale deeply as you straighten and reach over leg in both movements 2 and 3.

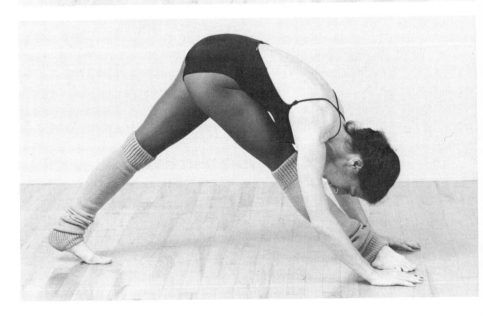

148

Seventeen ROLL-UP AND STRETCH

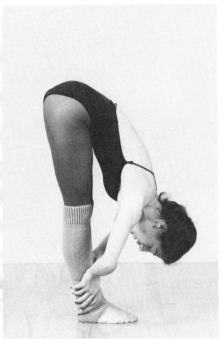

Starting position: Bring your legs together with both knees straight. Keep your upper torso stretched forward over your thighs.

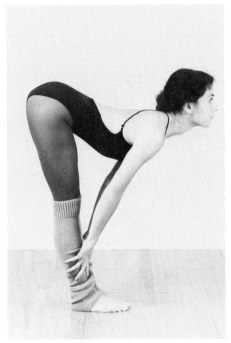

1. Grab your ankles and arch your back, lifting your head and chin up, for 4 counts.

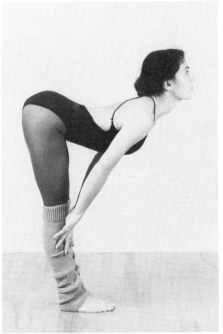

2. Then reach out with your chest even farther, arching your back as much as you can and reaching your buttocks toward the ceiling for 4 counts.

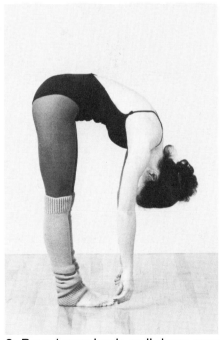

3. Round your back, pull down over your thighs.

Repeat movements 1, 2 and 3 once.

CONTINUED→

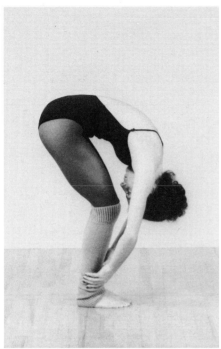

4. Round your back down over your thighs. Knees are bent. Let your arms and shoulders relax. Slowly roll up one vertebra at a time.

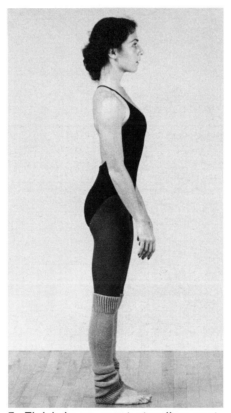

5. Finish in an erect standing position, stomach pulled in, buttocks tight, pulling up and out of your hips.

Breathing: Inhale, then exhale as you arch up. Inhale, then exhale as you round down.

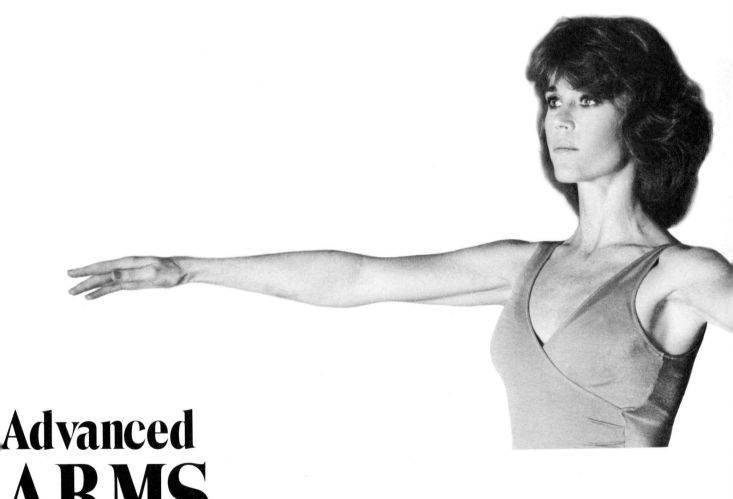

Advanced
ARMS

ARMS 4 MINUTES

Purpose: To strengthen, tone and render flexible every part of your arms, shoulders and chest.

Music:
Irene Cara—"Fame"/*Fame*
Irene Cara—"Red Light"/*Fame*
Kongas—"Gimme Some Lovin' "/*Africanism*
Karen Young—"Hot Shot"/*Hot Shot*
Dan Hartman—"Instant Replay"/*Instant Replay*
Paul Jabara—"Pleasure Island"/*Keeping Time*
Johnny Lee—"Lookin' for Love"/*Urban Cowboy*

One STRAIGHT ARM CIRCLES
Deltoids, trapezius

Starting position: Standing with feet together, buttocks tight, stomach pulled in, body pulled up, shoulders down.

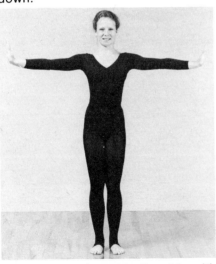 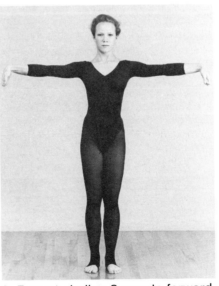 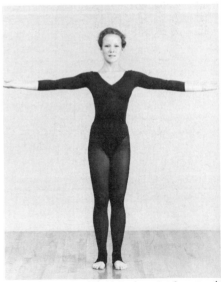

1. Arms straight out to the side with wrists flexed upward, heels of your hands pushing to opposite walls. Circle the arms forward 8 counts and back 8 counts, being sure to keep the shoulders from hunching up. The circling motion is with the entire arm from the shoulder. Make the circles as large as you can.

2. Repeat circling 8 counts forward, 8 counts back with wrists flexed downward, backs of hands pushing to side walls as hard as you can, knuckles folded under.

3. Repeat circling 8 counts forward, 8 counts back with palms facing the ceiling.

Breathing: Steady breathing

Two
SHOULDER RELEASE
To release deltoids

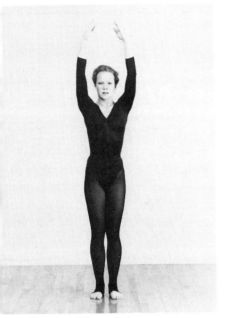

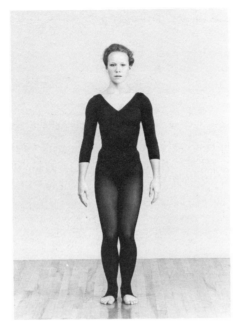

Starting position: Bring your arms down to your sides.

1. Swing your arms out to the side and over your head.

2. Swing your arms down to your sides as you bend your knees slightly.

These two movements are done to one count. Repeat for a total of 8 counts, straightening the knees as you do movement 1.

Breathing: Exhale as arms come down. Inhale as arms go up.

Three
ELBOW EXTENSIONS
Triceps

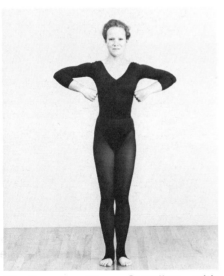

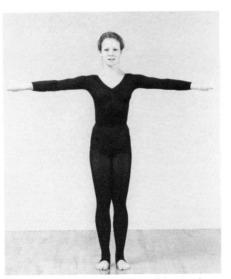

Starting position: Standing with knees straight, raise your elbows out to the side at shoulder height. Your lower arm is bent in toward your body, fists are clenched, palms facing the back wall.

Extend your lower arm (through a downward arc) out to shoulder height. Try not to move your shoulders or upper arms, and keep your fists clenched, palms facing back wall.

Return to starting position. Open and close your lower arms like this 10 times.

Breathing: Exhale as you extend arm from elbow. Inhale as you bring lower arm back to starting position.

Four
SHOULDER TWISTS
Deltoids, triceps

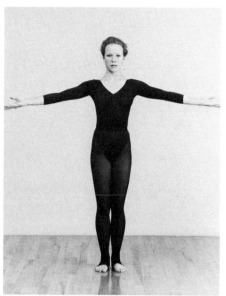 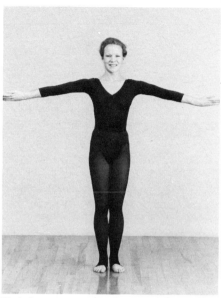

Starting position: Arms are extended straight to the side, shoulder height, palms up.

Rotate your arms forward from the shoulders, then release your arms backward from the shoulder, to starting position.

The two movements are done to one count. Do for 16 counts. Imagine you're turning a doorknob with each hand.

Be sure not to move anything but your arms. It's a small movement which should cause a burning sensation. Good! Go for it!

Breathing: Exhale as arm turns forward from shoulder. Inhale as arm turns back.

Five
SHOULDER RELEASE
To release deltoids

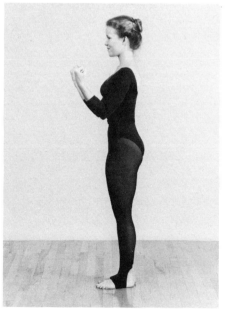 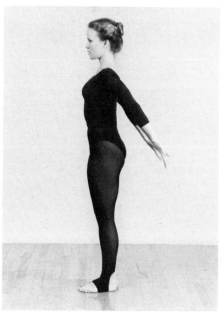

Starting position: Bring your arms in front of you, parallel to each other with elbows bent, fists clenched.

1. Keeping your arms close to your sides, swing them down and behind you as far as you can without moving your torso. The hands open, palms to back wall, at the end of the swing.

2. Then pull arms forward to starting position.

The swing back and pull forward are done to one count. Repeat for a total of 8 counts.

Breathing: Exhale as arms swing behind body. Inhale as arms pull forward.

Six
FLAT-BACK SCISSORS
Deltoids, triceps, trapezius

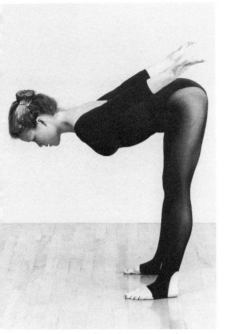

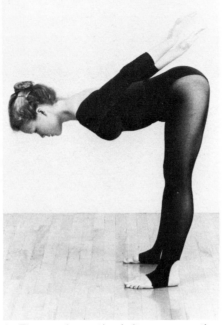

These two movements are done to one count.

Be sure to keep your elbows locked and your arms as high as possible. Scissor for 16 counts.

Breathing: Steady breathing

1. Reach over with a flat back and straight legs while you scissor your arms behind your back, crossing the right arm over the left.

2. Then scissor the left arm over the right.

Seven
THE OVERHEAD BRIDGE
Stretches deltoids, triceps, trapezius

Clasp your hands behind your back, let your head and back drop down as far as you can. Let your arms fall as far over your head as possible, stretching out your shoulders.

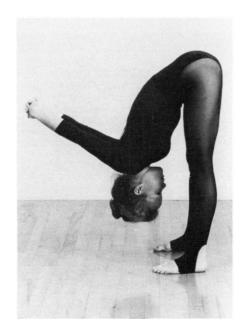

Breathing: Normal

Eight

BACK OF THE ARM EXTENSIONS
Triceps

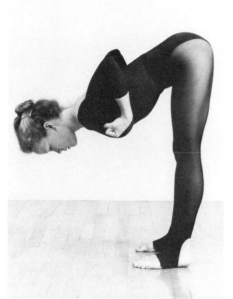

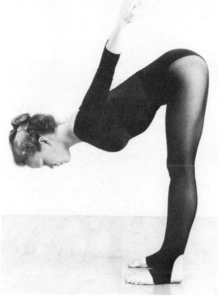

Starting position: With your feet a little more than hip distance apart, flatten your back and bend your elbows, arms close to your sides, fists held at the sides of your breasts.

Keeping your legs straight, extend your arms and hands straight up from your elbow as high as possible behind your back, opening your hands and stretching through the fingers. Then bend arms in again as in starting position.

The two movements are done to one count. Repeat for a total of 20 counts. Be sure to keep arms close to your sides.

Breathing: Exhale as arms extend behind body. Inhale as arms bend in.

Nine

PULLING WEEDS
Biceps

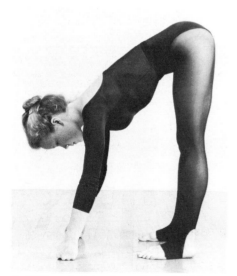

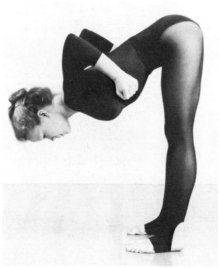

1. With a flat back and straight legs, reach forward with your arms as though you were grabbing weeds.

2. Now quickly, pull your arms back with your elbows bent behind you, fists clenched, as though you were angrily pulling up the weeds.

These two movements are done to one count. Repeat for a total of 10 counts.

Breathing: Exhale as you pull arms up. Inhale as you reach forward.

Ten

SCISSORS
Pectorals

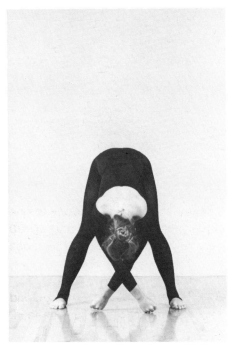

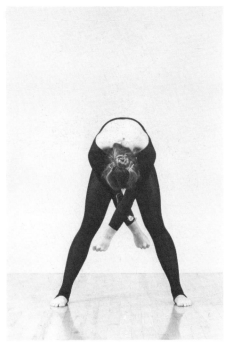

Starting position: Standing with feet a little more than hip distance apart, let your body hang over with arms crossed.

1. As you roll up, cross the left arm over the right arm, then the right arm over the left arm, in a scissoring motion.

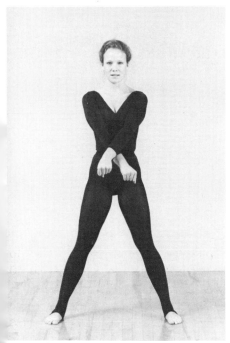

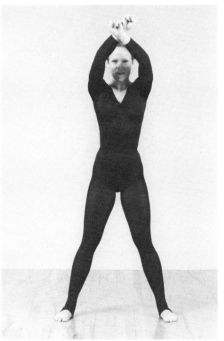

2. When you've rolled up to a standing position, continue to scissor the arms upward.

3. Scissor the arms up over your head, then scissor them back down again, as you remain standing up straight.

Take 8 counts to bring the arms up and 8 counts to bring them back down.

Try to open the arms as wide as you can before you scissor them and try not to move the rest of the body.

This is an excellent exercise for the pectoral muscles, which support the breasts.

Breathing: Steady breathing

Eleven

ARM STRETCHES
To release pectorals

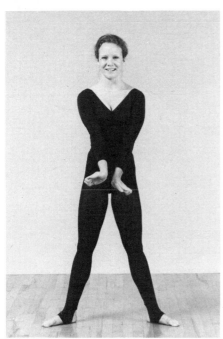

Starting position: Stand with arms straight and held in front of you, both hands flexed, knuckles folded under.

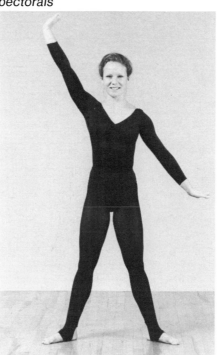

1. Swing your right arm up and back over your head while your left arm swings down and back, opening your chest in a diagonal pull.

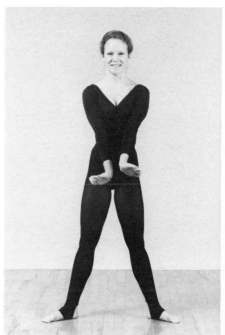

2. Bring arms together as in starting position. These two movements are done to one count. Repeat movements 1 and 2 (*i.e.,* do this for 2 counts to the right).

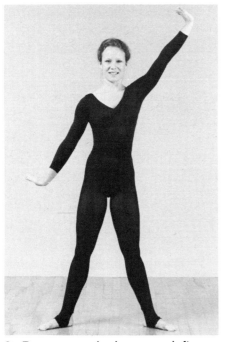

3. Reverse, swinging your left arm up and your right arm down and back.

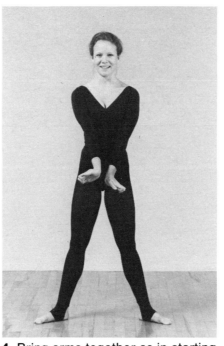

4. Bring arms together as in starting position. These two movements are done to one count. Repeat movements 3 and 4 (*i.e.,* do for 2 counts to the left).

Do the entire set twice, a total of 8 counts.

Breathing: Exhale as both arms swing out. Inhale as they meet in front of you.

SHAKE YOUR ARMS OUT.

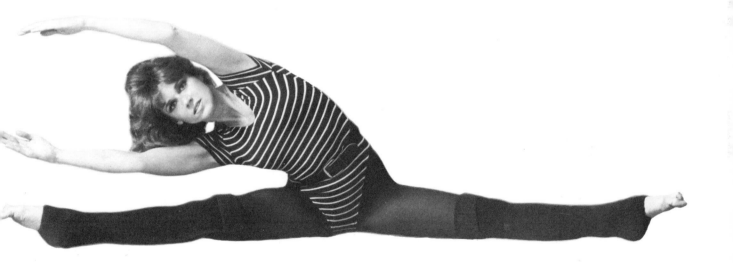

Advanced
WAIST

WAIST

7 MINUTES (including floor work)

Purpose: To reduce the fatty deposits at the waistline, tone, shape and strengthen the waist and back muscles.

Music:

Jacksons—"Can You Feel It"/*Triumph*
Roberta Kelly—"Oh Happy Day"/*Gettin' the Spirit*
Roberta Kelly—"To My Father's House"/*Gettin' the Spirit*
Isaac Hayes—"Don't Let Go"/*Don't Let Go*
Eddie Rabbitt—"I Love a Rainy Night"/*Horizon*
Donna Summer—"Hot Stuff"/*Bad Girls*
Donna Summer—"MacArthur Park"/*Live and More*
Pattie Brooks—"Don't Make Me Wait"/*Love Shook*
Amii Stewart—"Light My Fire"/*Knock on Wood*

One

SIDE PULLS
Intercostals, obliques

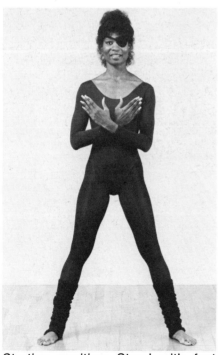 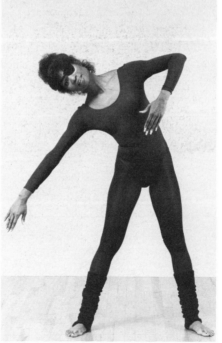 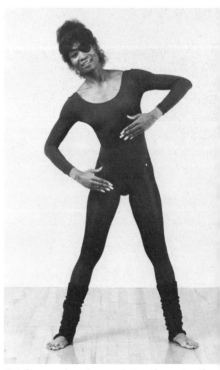

Starting position: Stand with feet apart, stomach pulled in, buttocks tight, hands in front of your torso, palms facing your body. Imagine you are standing between two sheets of glass. If you lean forward, you'll break the glass.

1. Pull over to the right, reaching down and out with your right arm while your left elbow bends upward as far as it can go. You should feel a pull up the left side of your body. Let your head relax to the right. Keep your left shoulder back and your hips forward.

2. Come back up into the starting position. This down and up movement is done to one count. Do 40 counts to the right.

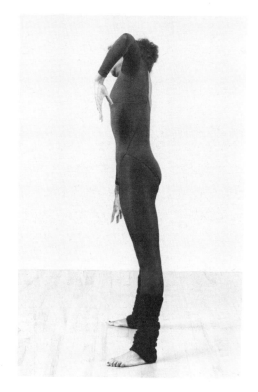

3. Repeat 40 counts to the left, reaching down with your left arm and up with your bent right elbow. (Increase to 60 in each direction as you gain strength.) Be sure to keep your right shoulder back and your hips forward.

This is probably the most effective exercise I've found for slimming the waist, but in order to get the most out of it, you must go directly to the side and not let your upper torso pull forward.

Breathing: Exhale as you reach out. Inhale as you come up.

Two

MORE SIDE PULLS
Intercostals, obliques

1. Pull over to the right, extending your left arm directly over your ear, your right arm curved in front of you. Bounce gently for 8 counts, being sure to keep your hips forward, weight evenly distributed on both feet and left shoulder back.

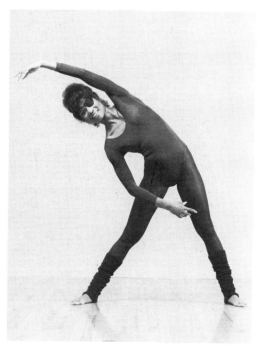

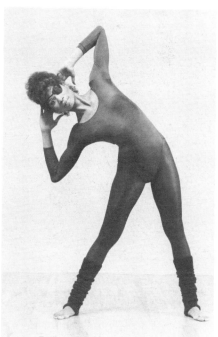

2. Place both hands behind your head and bounce gently to the right side for 8 counts. Don't let your elbows pull inward; keep them opened outward.

CONTINUED→

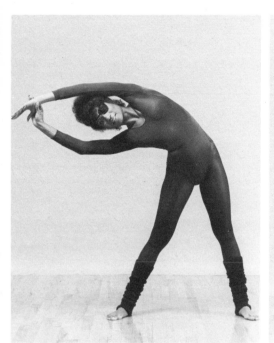

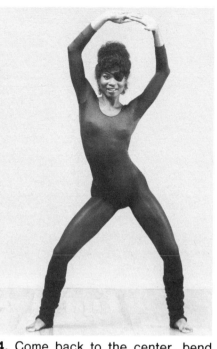

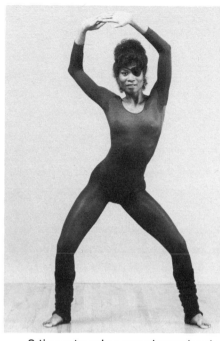

3. Reach both arms to the right, grab your left wrist with your right hand and pull over, pulsing gently for 8 counts.

4. Come back to the center, bend your knees, clasp hands and circle your hips and arms . . .

. . . 8 times to relax your lower back.

Repeat to the left, 8 counts in each position, ending with the hip and arm circles.

Breathing: Exhale as you reach out. Inhale as you release between reaches.

Three SIDE-TO-SIDE
Intercostals, obliques

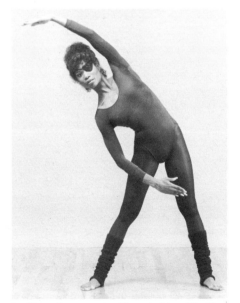

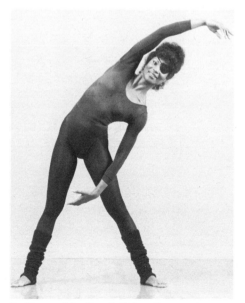

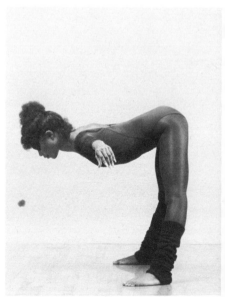

1. Reach over to the right with the left arm, the right arm curved in front of you, and bounce to the side twice, taking one count for each bounce-release.

2. Repeat to the left for 2 counts.

3. Open both arms out at shoulder height and bounce over with flat back and straight legs for 2 counts.

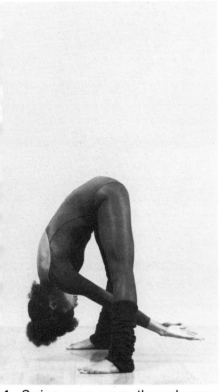

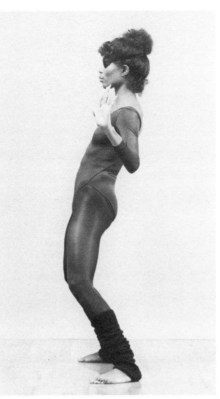

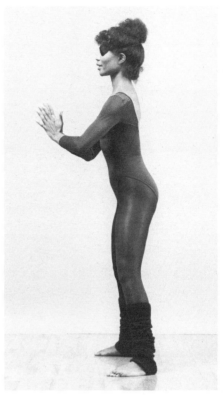

4. Swing your arms through your straight legs and bounce for 2 counts.

5. Swing up and bounce your hips forward with slightly bent knees for 2 counts . . .

. . . clapping in between the forward bounces.

Do the entire sequence a total of three times.

Breathing: Steady breathing

Four
WAIST TWISTS
Intercostals, obliques

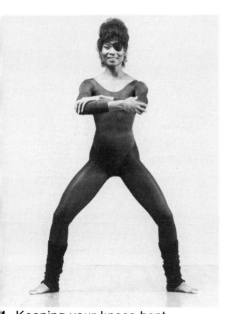

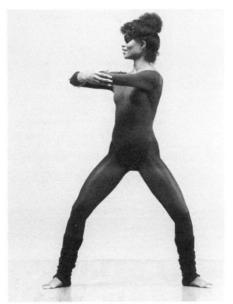

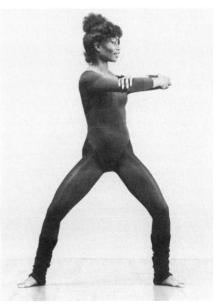

1. Keeping your knees bent . . .

. . . grab your elbows and twist to the right 4 counts looking over your right shoulder.

2. Repeat to the left 4 counts.

Repeat 4 counts to each side.

CONTINUED→

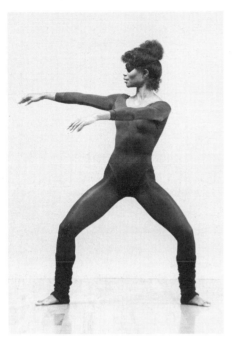

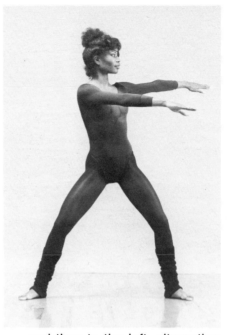

Keep your arms at shoulder height during these swings.

Breathing: Steady breathing

3. Let go of your elbows and swing your open arms to the right . . .

. . . and then to the left, alternating right and left for a total of 8 swings.

Five

ELBOW LUNGE
Intercostals, obliques

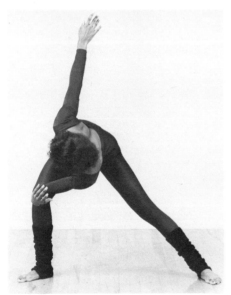

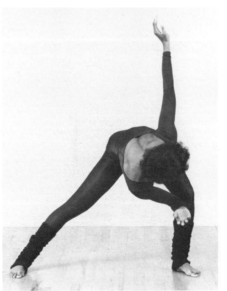

Alternate to the right and left for a total of 8 counts.

1. As you finish your last open-arm swing, simply lunge to the right, bending your right knee and straightening the left, reaching your left elbow to your right knee. Let your right arm swing up behind you, twist and look up at the ceiling. This is done to one count.

2. Repeat to the left, reaching your right elbow to the left knee for one count, twisting as you do to look at the ceiling.

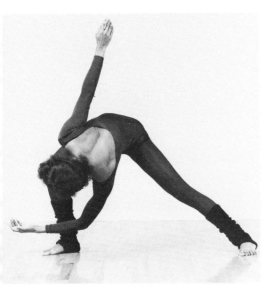

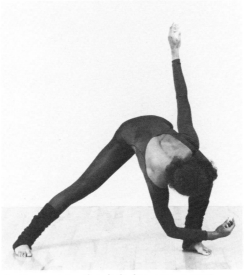

Breathing: Steady breathing

3. Now lunge lower and reach your left elbow to your right ankle, swing your right arm behind you, twist and look at the ceiling for one count.

4. Repeat to the left for one count.

Alternate to the right and left for a total of 8 counts.

Now repeat both the elbow-to-knee, elbow-to-ankle sequences one more time, for 8 counts each.

Six

HIP RELEASE
To release upper inner thigh

Starting position: Bend your knees into a squatting position, bring your hands between your knees and place them behind your feet. You'll find your inner knees are resting on your elbows, which should stretch your inner thighs open.

Small bounces with your buttocks for 16 counts.

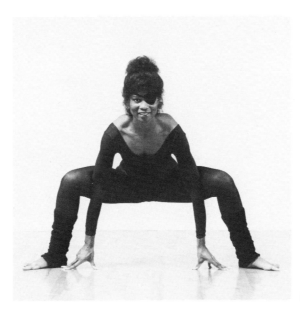

Breathing: Normal breathing

Seven ROLL-UP

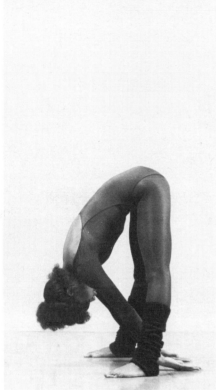

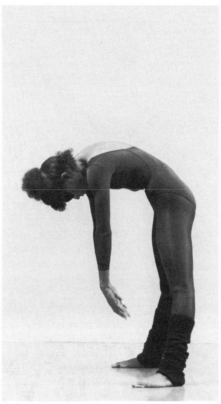

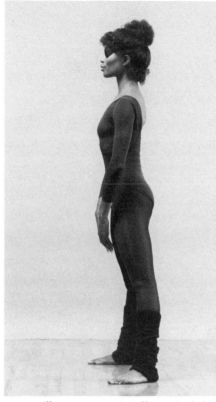

Starting position: Keep your hands behind your feet as you straighten your knees.

Let your arms and head hang limp like a rag doll and slowly roll up, one vertebra at a time . . .

. . . until you are standing straight.

Breathing: Normal

Waist exercises continue on the floor.
Get a mat, towel, blanket or whatever you need to have a soft padding to work out on.

Eight WAIST AND INNER THIGH STRETCH
Intercostals, obliques

Starting position: Sitting on the floor, open your legs as wide as you can without straining the tendons along your inner thighs. Point your toes.

1. Pull over to the right side trying to aim your ear to your leg. Your left arm is pulling directly over to the right while your right arm is gracefully curved in front of you. Bounce down gently for 8 counts.

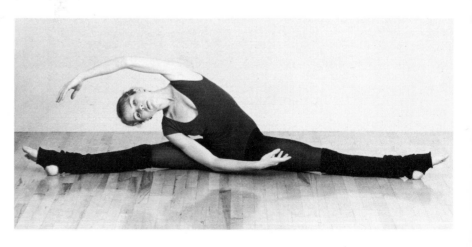

. Repeat this movement to the left
ide, bouncing down for 8 counts.

Repeat, alternating sides, for 6
ounts, then 4 counts, and twice for
? counts. Then do 10 singles, side to
ide.

Vhen you are pulling to one side, try
o keep the opposite hip on the floor
ind be sure to go straight to the
ide.

Breathing: Exhale as you reach; in-
ale as you release before reaching.

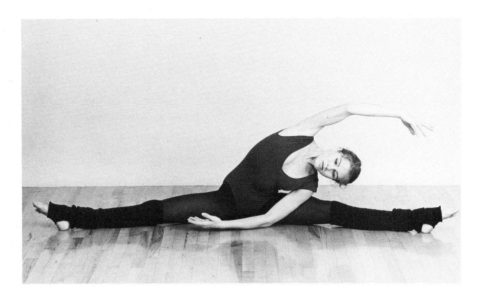

Nine

CHEST-TO-KNEE STRETCH
Intercostals, obliques

. Place your hands on each side of
your right leg and stretch down,
eaching your chest toward your
knee. Bounce gently for 8 counts.

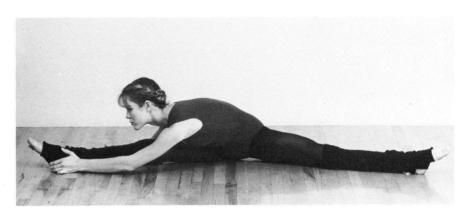

. With your hands on the floor in
ront of you, stretch out of your hip
ind "walk" yourself around . . .

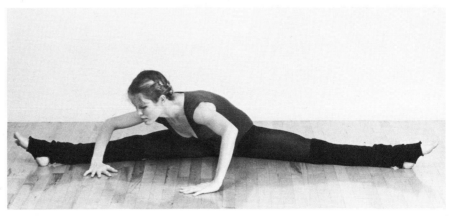

CONTINUED→

. . . to the left. Keep your torso as low as possible to the floor. Take 4 counts to get to the left side.

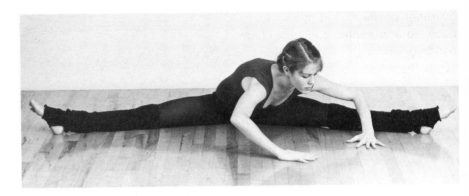

3. Place your hands on each side of your left leg and stretch down, reaching your chest toward your knee. Bounce gently for 8 counts.

Repeat once to each side.

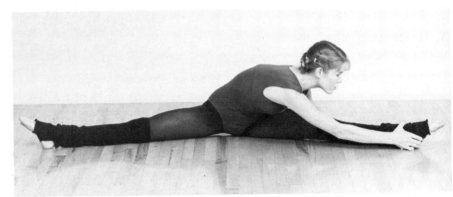

4. "Walk" to the center again and gently bounce down as low as you can with your hands on the floor in front of you for support and your toes pointed. Bounce for 8 counts.

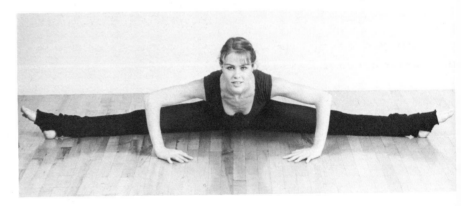

5. Try to open your legs a little wider, flex your feet and bounce gently for another 8 counts.

Breathing: Steady breathing

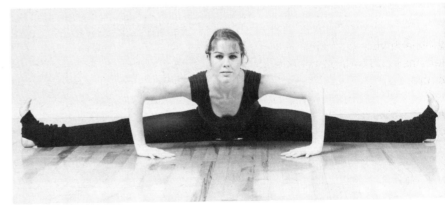

Ten

SIDE ELBOW BEND
Intercostals, obliques

Starting position: Lift your torso back up into center position, place hands behind your head with elbows out to the side.

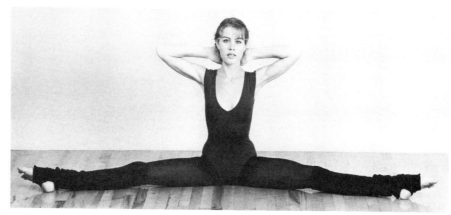

1. Reach your right elbow out to your right knee and . . .

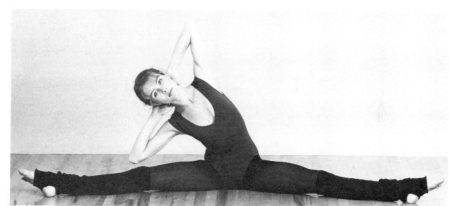

. . . come back to center. These two movements are done to one count.

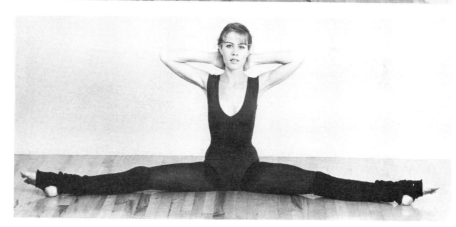

2. Reach your left elbow out to your left knee and return to center for one count.

Alternate sides for a total of 10 counts.

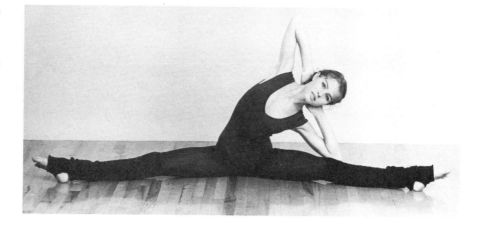

Breathing: Exhale as elbow touches knee. Inhale as you come to center.

Eleven

THE KILLER STRETCH
Hamstrings

Starting position: Bring your legs together and sit up straight. Grab your toes and flex your feet so hard your heels are lifted off the floor.

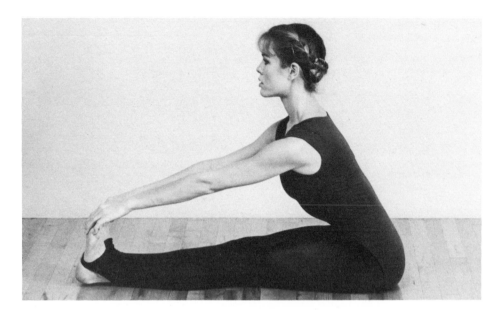

Pull your torso down over your legs as far as you can go. Try to keep your heels lifted off the floor while you strive to touch your elbows to the floor. Hold for 10 counts.

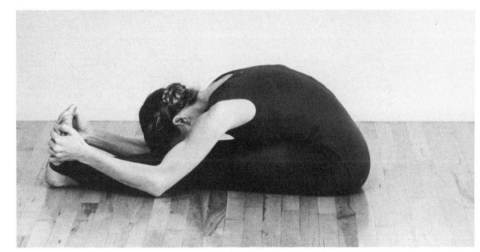

Keep pulling your heels off the floor.

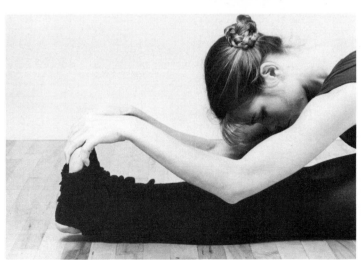

Breathing: Inhale deeply to begin, then exhale deeply as you pull down, to relax and lengthen the stretch.

Shake your legs out by slapping them against the floor a few times.

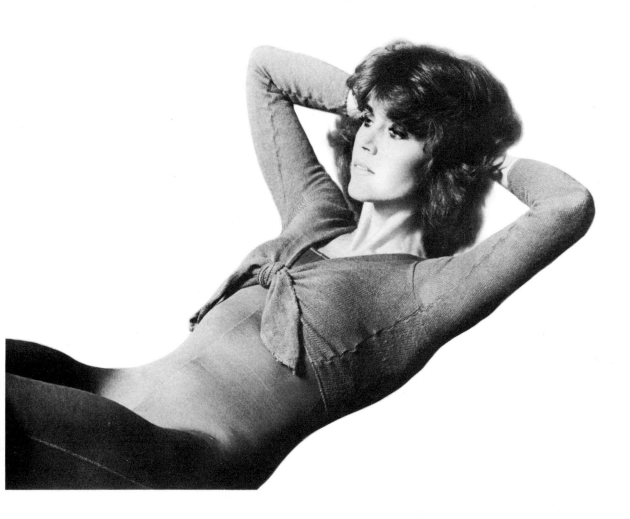

Advanced
ABDOMINALS

ABDOMINALS 7 MINUTES

Purpose: To burn away the fatty deposits around your stomach, to slim, tone and strengthen the upper and lower abdominal muscles.

Music:

Linda Clifford—"Bridge Over Troubled Water"/*Let Me Be Your Woman*
Blondie—"Call Me"/*American Gigolo*
Irene Cara—"Fame"/*Fame*
Irene Cara—"Red Light"/*Fame*
Sylvester—"You Make Me Feel"/*Step 2*
Sylvester—"Dance Disco Heat"/*Step 2*
Voyage—"Souvenirs"/*Night at Studio 54*
Musique—"In the Bush"/*Night at Studio 54*
D. C. LaRue—"Hot Jungle Drums & Voodoo Rhythm"/*Night at Studio 54*
Evelyn "Champagne" King—"Shame"/*Smooth Talk*
Evelyn "Champagne" King—"Nobody Knows"/*Smooth Talk*
Gloria Gaynor—"I Will Survive"/*Love Tracks*

If you're using weights, this is the time to put them on.

Note of caution: **You must be careful to keep your stomach pulled in as you do these exercises, so as not to develop a protruding abdomen.**

One

SIT-UPS
Lower abdominals

Starting position: Lie on your back, knees bent, feet and knees parallel about a foot apart, feet flat on floor, hands behind your head with your elbows out to the sides.

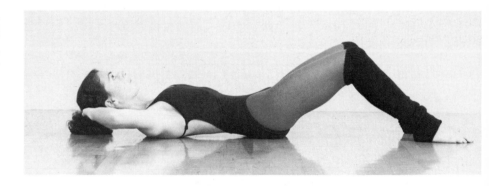

1. Lift your head and upper back off the floor as high as you can, using your abdominal muscles, not your arms. Keep your elbows back.

2. Lower a little but do not touch the floor.

Do these lifts, combining movements 1 and 2, 40 times. Try to come higher each time. Go for the burn!

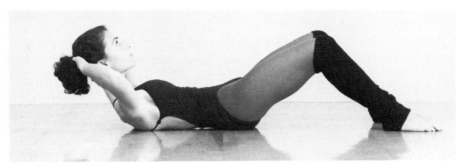

Breathing: Exhale as you lift up, inhale as you lower.

Two

THROUGH LEG REACHES
Upper and lower abdominals

Starting position: Turn out your feet slightly, opening the space between your knees. Extend your arms back over your head.

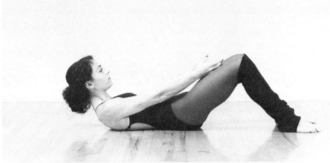

1. Reach your arms forward through your knees, lifting your head and shoulders off the floor.

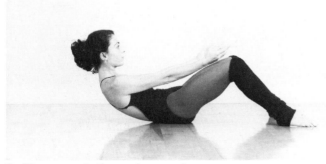

3. Then reach through your knees, lifting your upper torso off the floor. Pull through, releasing slightly between pulls, 30 times.

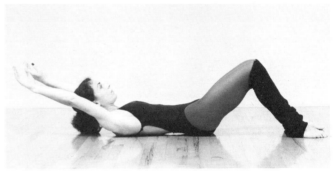

2. Swing your arms back toward the floor again, taking care not to let your arms drop behind your ears. Lower your head and shoulders toward the floor but don't let them touch the floor.

Lift and lower, repeating movements 1 and 2, 20 times.

Breathing: Exhale as you reach through, inhale as you lower.

Three

KNEES TO CHEST
To release abdominals

With head and shoulders down on the floor, hug your knees tightly in to your chest for 10 counts. This position is especially soothing and beneficial for the female organs.

Breathing: Normal

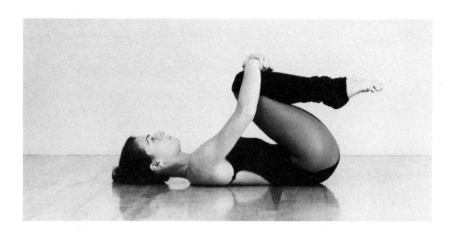

Four

CLIMB ROPE
Lower abdominals

1. With knees bent, feet and knees parallel, lift your upper torso off the floor and reach up with the left arm.

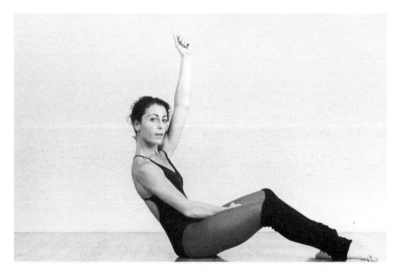

2. Reach up with the right arm as you pull down with the left. It should feel as if you're pulling yourself up a rope.

The right and left reach and pull are done to one count. Repeat for a total of 20 counts.

Keep your torso low enough to work your abdominals to their maximum.

Breathing: Exhale as you pull down; take a breath before your next pull.

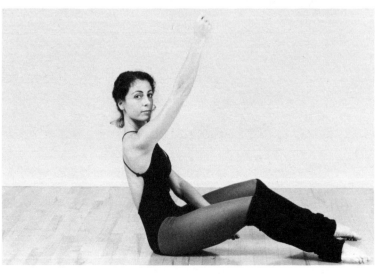

Five

KNEES TO CHEST
To release abdominals

Head and shoulders on the floor, hug your knees tightly in to your chest for 10 counts.

Breathing: Normal

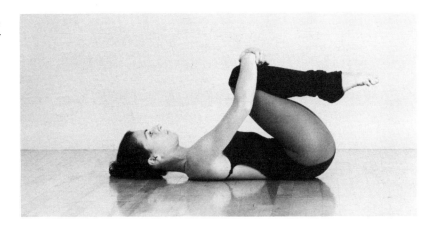

Six

THE BICYCLE
Obliques, lower abdominals

1. Place your hands behind your head and extend the right leg straight out, a few inches off the floor, toes pointed. Bend your left knee in to your chest, reaching your right elbow to touch your left knee.

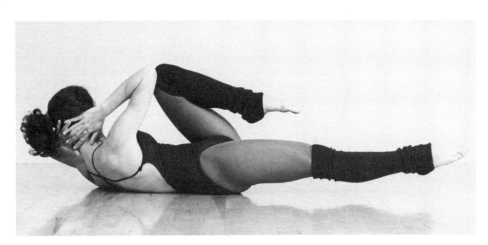

2. Switch sides, extending the left leg out with toe pointed. Bend the right knee in and touch the left elbow to the right knee.

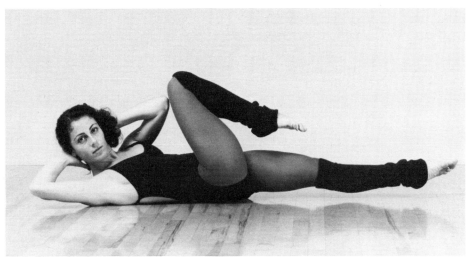

These two movements, right and left, are done to one count. Repeat for a total of 16 counts with toes pointed,

CONTINUED→

. . . then do 16 times with feet flexed.

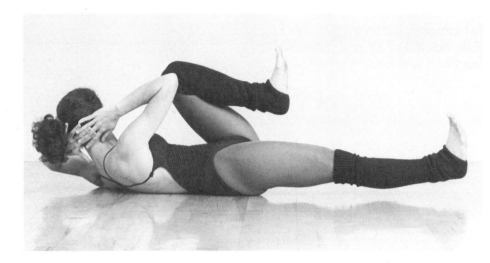

Be sure to straighten the leg as you extend it, and keep it close to the floor.

Breathing: Steady breathing

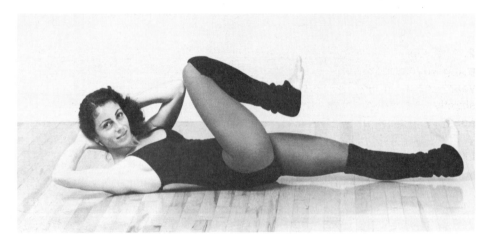

Seven   KNEES TO CHEST
To release abdominals

Hug your knees tightly in to your chest for 10 counts.

Breathing: Normal

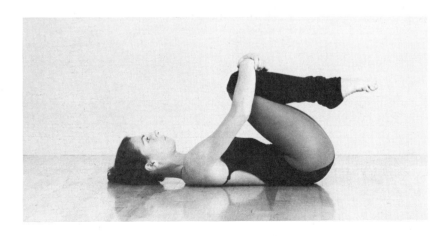

Eight

EXTENDED LEG SIT-UPS
Lower and upper abdominals

1. Extend your legs straight up with toes pointed, hands behind your head with your elbows back.

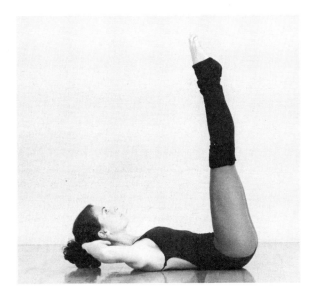

2. Lift your head and upper torso using your abdominal muscles, not your arms, then release back slightly but don't touch the floor again.

Lift and release 30 times.

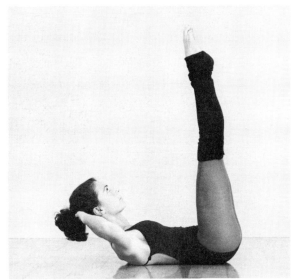

3. Lift up even farther, extending your arms past your lifted legs. Lift like this, releasing back slightly between lifts, for 30 counts.

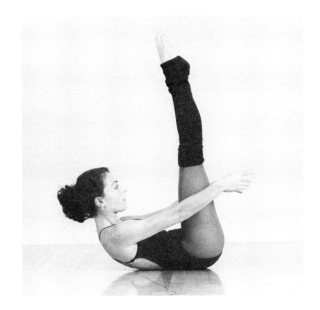

Breathing: Exhale as you lift up, inhale as you release back.

Nine

KNEES TO CHEST
To release abdominals

Hug your knees tightly in to your chest for 10 counts.

Breathing: Normal

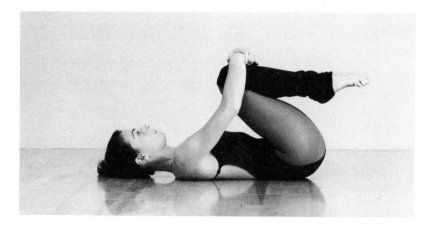

Ten

EXTENDED SCISSOR KICKS
Upper and lower abdominals, inner thigh, quadriceps

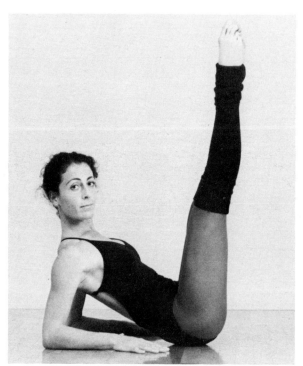

Starting position: Extend your legs straight up with your toes pointed. Come up onto your elbows, palms of your hands flat on the floor.

1. Scissor-kick your straight legs, right leg over left, left leg over right, lowering them as you scissor for 8 counts.

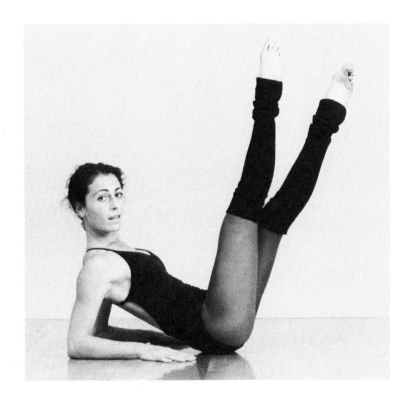

2. Continue scissor-kicking with your legs a few inches off the floor with toes pointed for 16 counts.

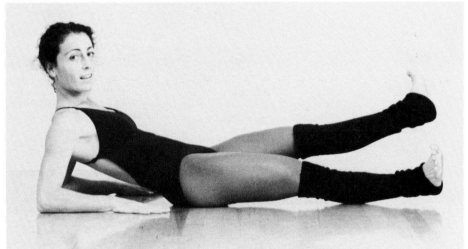

3. Scissor-kick for 16 more counts with feet flexed.

Breathing: Steady breathing

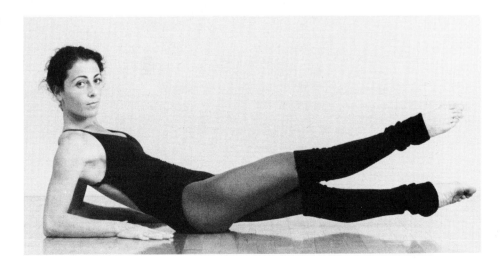

Eleven KNEES TO CHEST
To release abdominals

Hug your knees tightly in to your chest for 10 counts.

Breathing: Normal

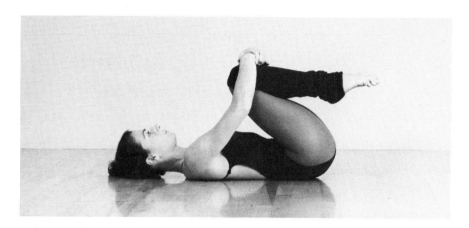

Twelve STOMACH RELEASE
To release abdominals and lower back

1. Swing your knees over to the right side and your arms to the left.

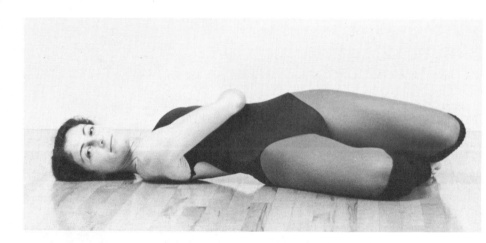

2. Swing your knees over to the left side and your arms to the right.

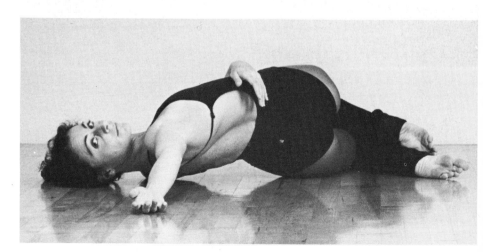

Repeat once to each side.

Breathing: Normal

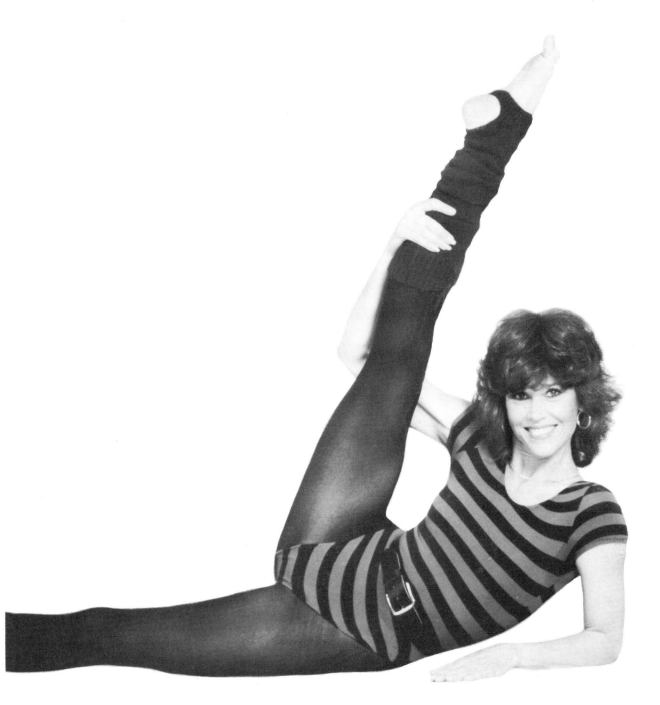

Advanced
LEGS AND HIPS

LEGS AND HIPS 10 MINUTES

Purpose:

To burn off the fatty deposits, tone and strengthen the muscles on the sides of the hips and thighs, the troublesome inner thighs and the back of the hips. These are the best, most effective exercises I've ever found for these problem areas.

Music:

Dolly Parton—"Baby I'm Burnin' "/*Heartbreaker*
Fleetwood Mac—"Dreams"/*Rumours*
Brothers Johnson—"Stomp"/*Light Up the Night*
Eddie Rabbitt—"I Love a Rainy Night"/*Horizon*
Chic—"Le Freak"/*C'est Chic*
Taste of Honey—"Boogie Oogie Oogie"/*Taste of Honey*
Jacksons—"Shake Your Body Down"/*Destiny*
Paul Jabara—"Shut Out"/*Perils of Paul*
Linda Clifford—"One of Those Songs"/*Let Me Be Your Woman*

One

LEG LIFTS TO THE SIDE
Gluteus medius, gluteus minimus, tensor fasciae latae

Starting position: Lie on your left side, up on your left elbow, palms flat on the floor. Extend both legs straight out on a line with your upper body.

1. With toes pointed, lift your right leg up.

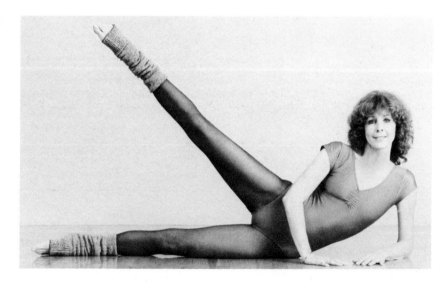

2. Lower your right leg but don't let it touch your bottom leg.

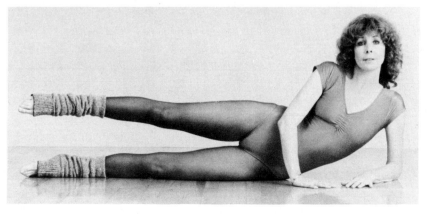

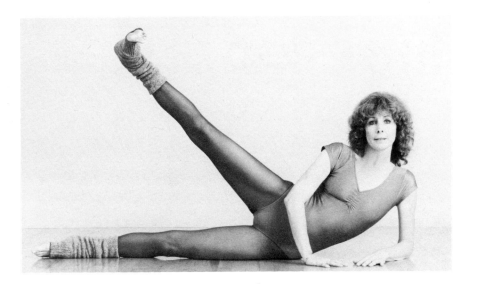

Do this movement 15 times with your toes pointed.

Repeat 15 times with your toes flexed.

Breathing: Exhale as leg lifts up, inhale as leg lowers.

Two

KNEE IN, LEG UP
Gluteus medius, gluteus minimus, tensor fasciae latae

1. Bend your right knee in to your body.

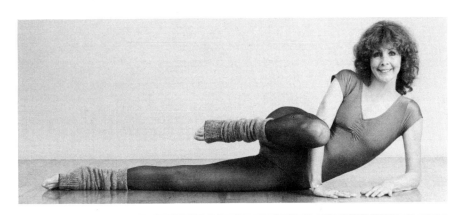

2. Extend your right leg straight out again, on a line with your left leg.

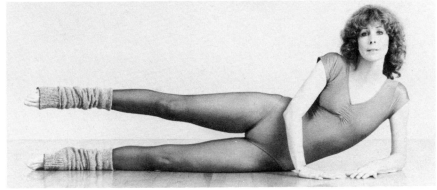

3. Lift your right leg straight up.

These three movements are done to one count. Repeat for a total of 10 counts.

Breathing: Exhale as leg extends, inhale as knee bends in.

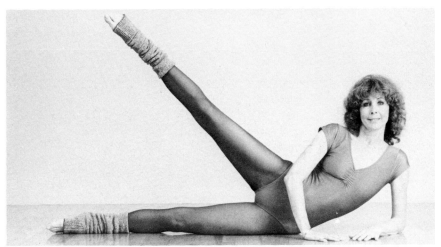

Three

CROSSOVERS

Gluteus maximus, medius, minimus, tensor fasciae latae and quadriceps

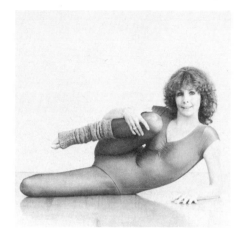

1. Bend your bottom leg, trying to align your thigh with your upper body. Grab your right knee with your right hand and pull your knee in to your chest.

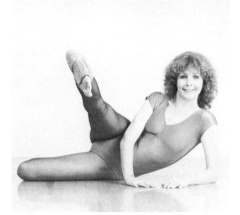

2. Extend your right leg straight out from your body, at a right angle to your left thigh. Turn your toes down so that your heel is higher than your toes.

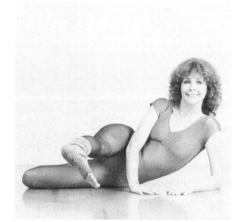

3. Lower your right leg to within a few inches of the floor.

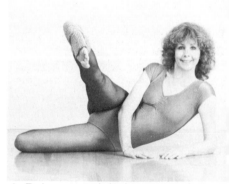

4. Raise your right leg up again.

Do these movements 15 times slowly and 30 times double-time.

Be sure to move the leg from the hip. Don't let the knee bend and, most emphatically, do not move the rest of the body. This is not an easy exercise and, as you begin to tire, there will be a tendency to raise and lower your leg by throwing your hips into it. Try feeling there's a wall against your back and you cannot rock your hips back.

Go for the burn! You'll like the results.

Breathing: Exhale as leg lowers, inhale as leg raises.

Four

BACK LEG LIFTS
Gluteus maximus, hamstrings

Starting position: Roll over so that your hips and chest are facing the floor. Come up on your left elbow and reach your right arm out in front of you. Extend both legs, knees straight, toes pointed. Cross the right leg over the left.

Lift your right leg as high as you can with toe pointed. Release it a little but don't let it drop too low. This is a small movement, lifting your leg from a lifted position. It will also strengthen your back.

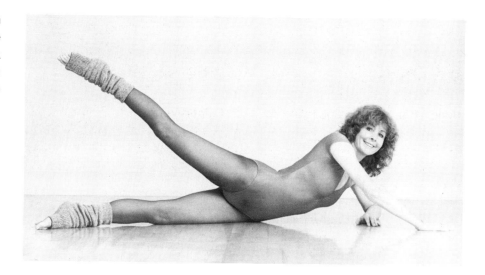

Do 20 counts with toes pointed and 20 counts with foot flexed.

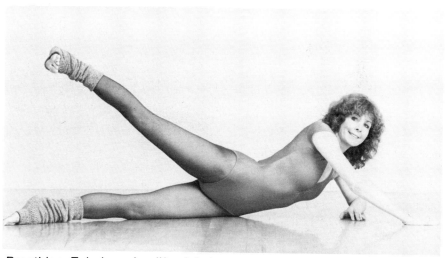

Breathing: Exhale as leg lifts, inhale as it releases.

Five

QUAD STRETCH
Stretches quadriceps

1. After the final back leg lift, reach around with your right hand and grab your right foot, stretching it in to your buttocks.

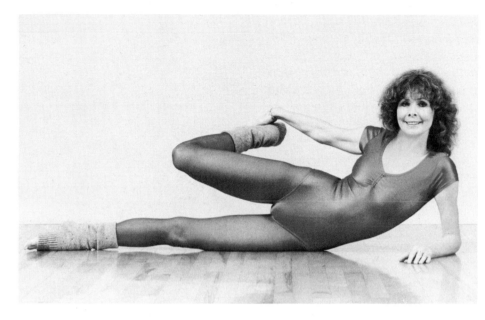

2. Then roll over onto your back with arms extended to the sides and your right leg bent under you. Lie in this position for 8 counts, pushing your right knee down and your right hip up. Feel the stretch up the front of your thigh.

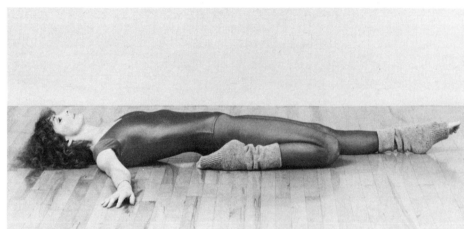

Breathing: Normal

Six

SCISSOR LIFTS

Inner thigh; adductor magnus, gracilis, pectineus

Starting position: Come back up onto your left buttock, resting on your left elbow.

1. Hold the ankle of your right leg with your right hand, toes pointed as you . . .

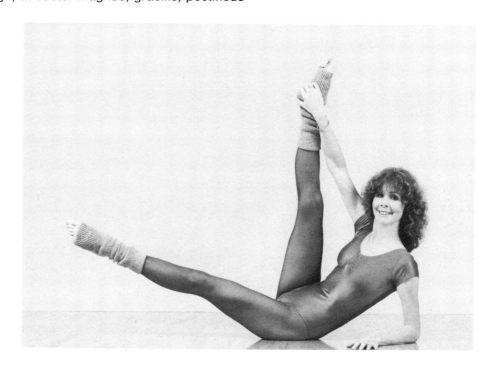

2. . . . lift your left leg up to meet your right leg and lower it.

Do this 10 times.

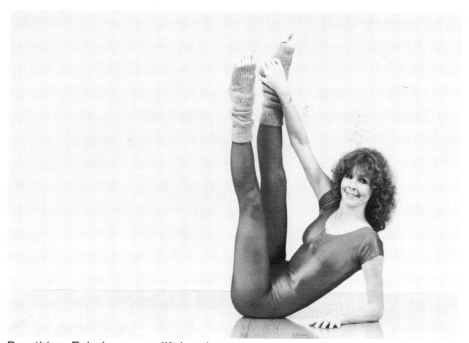

Breathing: Exhale as you lift leg; inhale as you lower it.

Seven

INNER THIGH LIFTS

Adductor magnus, adductor brevis, adductor longus, gracilis, pectineus

Starting position: Remain up on your left elbow. Grab your right foot with your right hand and bring it in front of your left leg which is extended an inch off the floor with toes pointed.

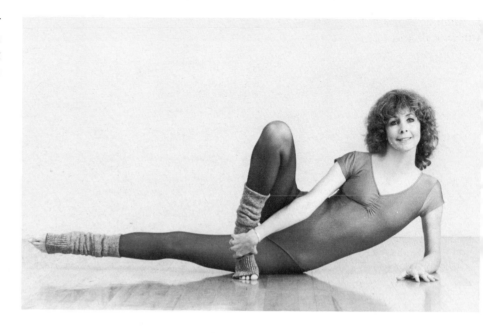

1. Lift your left leg, lowering it slightly between lifts, for 15 counts with toes pointed.

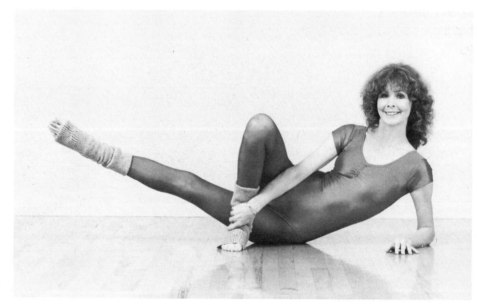

. Repeat, same leg, for 15 counts
with foot flexed.

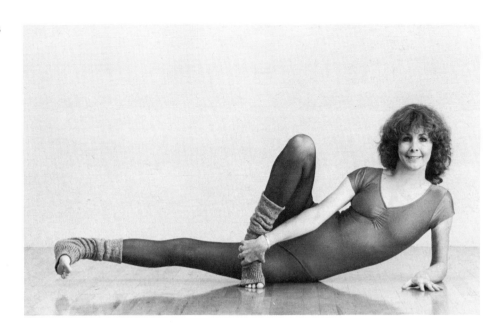

Be sure your left leg is turned out so
that the inner thigh is facing the ceiling.

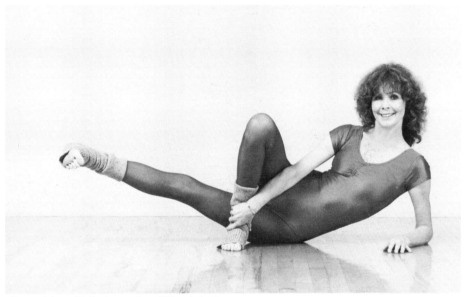

Breathing: Exhale as leg lifts, inhale
as it lowers between lifts.

Eight

HIP RELEASE
Stretches gluteus maximus

Starting position: Sit cross-legged on the floor, right foot in front of the left foot.

Round down over your bent legs and hold for 10 counts, then roll back up.

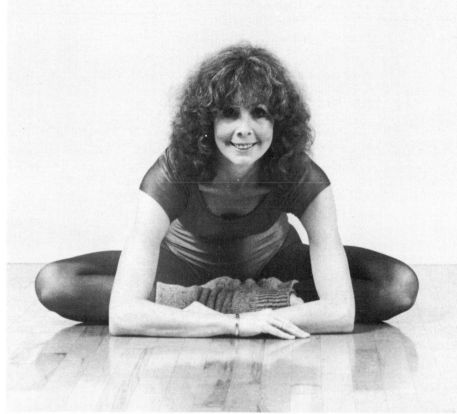

Breathing: Normal

Now you will repeat the entire sequence of leg and hip exercises (Exercises One through Eight) to the other side.

Music:

It is not necessary, but if you want to change the music for the final leg and hip sequence, here are some suggestions:

Kenny Loggins—''Whenever I Call You Friend''/*Nightwatch*
Melissa Manchester—''Whenever I Call You Friend''/*Manchester, Melissa*
Eddie Rabbitt—''Drivin' My Life Away''/*Horizon*
Cliff Richard—''Dreaming''/*I'm No Hero*
Jimmy Buffett—''Biloxi''/*Changes in Latitudes, Changes in Attitudes*

Nine

ROVER'S REVENGE
Gluteus maximus, medius, minimus, tensor fasciae latae, sartorius

Starting position: On your hands and knees, weight evenly distributed, back flat, stomach pulled in, head up.

1. Lift your right knee out to the side. Knee is bent and lifted to hip height, thigh parallel to the floor.

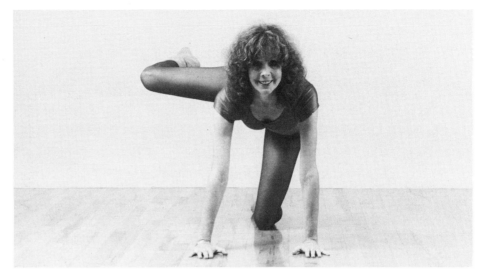

2. Lower your right knee down again but don't touch the floor. Lifting and lowering the knee are done to one count.

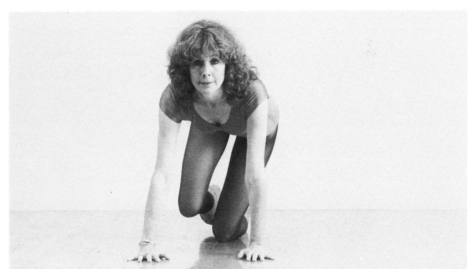

Repeat for a total of 30 counts. Try not to move the hips as you lift your knee. As you gain strength, increase to 50 counts.

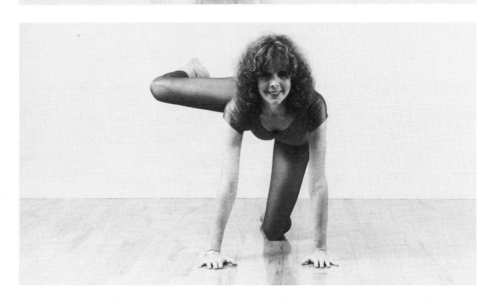

Breathing: Exhale as knee lifts, inhale as it lowers.

Ten

BACK LEG EXTENSIONS
Hamstrings

1. Extend the right leg straight behind you with toes pointed and lift it as high as you can 10 times, releasing it down slightly between lifts. Be sure your head is lifted and your back arched. Besides working the back of your hip, this exercise will also strengthen your back and make it more flexible.

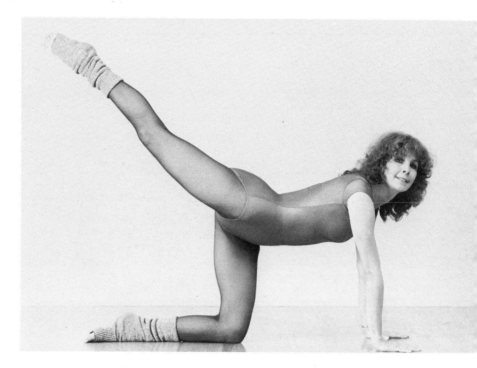

2. Repeat for 10 counts with foot flexed.

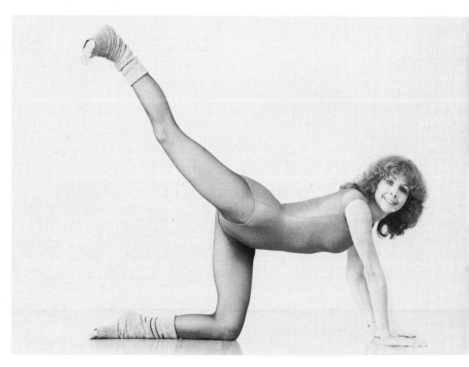

3. Contract your right knee in to your chest as you round your back and pull your head down. (Careful not to bump your nose with your knee!)

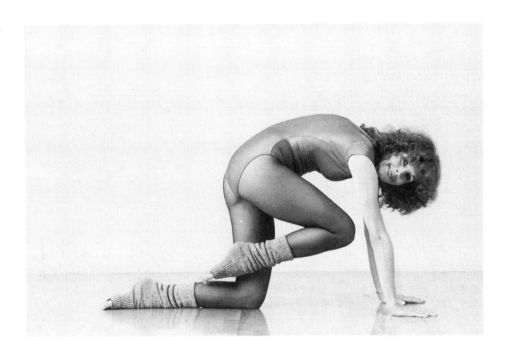

4. Swing your right leg back out and up again, lifting your head and arching your back.

These two movements in and out (3 and 4) are done to one count. Repeat for a total of 10 counts.

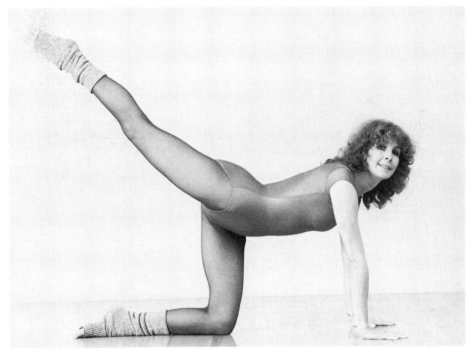

Breathing: Exhale as leg lifts, inhale as it releases.

Eleven DONKEY KICKS
Biceps femoris

1. As you swing your right leg up for the last time, leave it up there, bend your knee, flex your foot and kick your foot in to your buttock like an ornery mule.

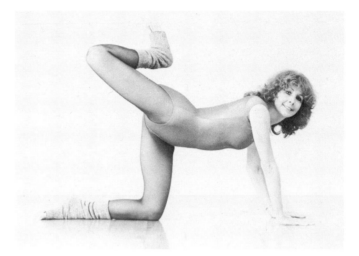

2. Extend your leg again.

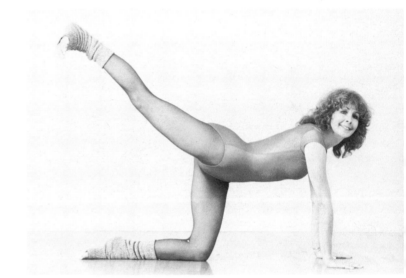

Repeat for a total of 20 counts, being sure to keep your knee higher than your hip.

While you do this, keep lifting that knee higher.

Breathing: Exhale as leg extends from knee, inhale as it kicks in.

Twelve PRAYING STRETCH
Stretches gluteus maximus

Sit back on your heels. Round down over your knees and extend your arms as far out in front of you as you can. Hold this position for 10 counts.

Breathing: Normal

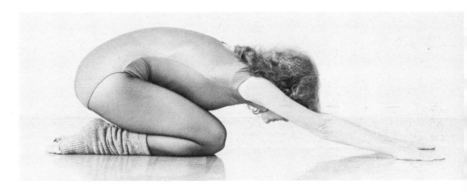

Now you will repeat Exercises Nine through Twelve to the left.

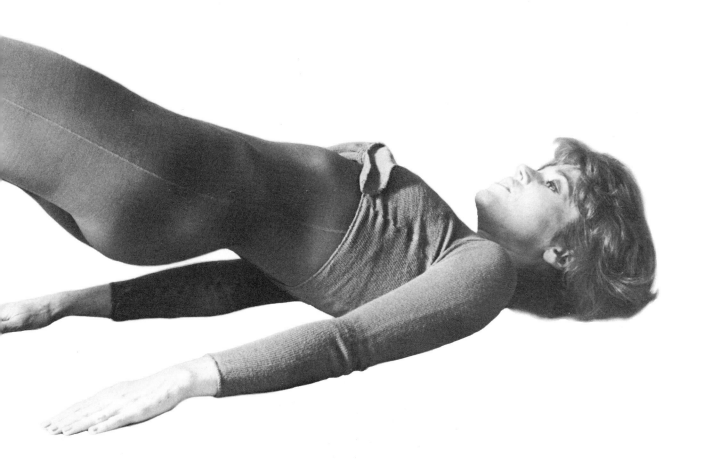

Advanced
BUTTOCKS

BUTTOCKS 4 MINUTES

Purpose:

To trim, tone and firm the buttocks (gluteus maximus, medius and minimus, biceps femoris). If you're eating properly this exercise will give you a smaller firmer butt, less apt to "fall," and those saddlebags will disappear.

Music:

Bob Seger—"Against the Wind"/*Against the Wind*
Sister Sledge—"We Are Family"/*We Are Family*
Michael Jackson—"Rock With You"/*Off the Wall*
Santana—"Stormy"/*Inner Secrets*
Cheryl Lynn—"Got to Be Real"/*Night at Studio 54*
Pointer Sisters—"Hypnotized"/*Energy*
Olivia Newton-John—"Totally Hot"/*Totally Hot*
Ralph McDonald—"Calypso"/*Saturday Night Fever*

One   BUTTOCKS LIFTS

Starting position: Lie on your back, feet parallel, a little more than hip distance apart, your arms lying alongside your body.

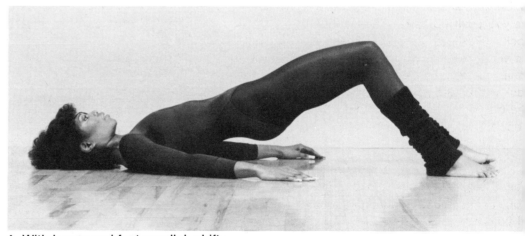

1. With knees and feet parallel, shift your weight onto your shoulders and lift your buttocks up . . .

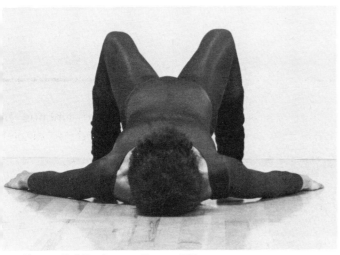

. . . then slightly lower them, lifting
and lowering for 30 counts.

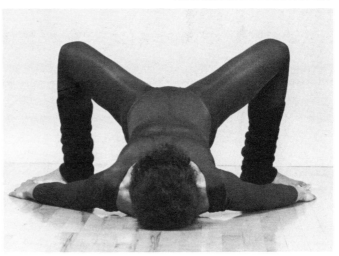

2. Turn your knees and feet out (let
them drop open) and continue lifting
your buttocks, lowering them
slightly between lifts, for 30 counts.

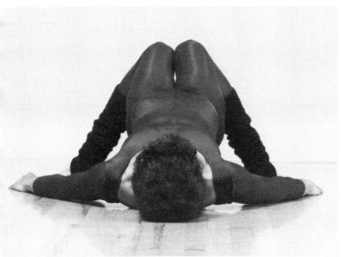

3. Bring your knees in till they touch,
as you push up hard with your buttocks. (Resist bringing your knees in
so you'll really work your outer and
inner thighs as well as your buttocks. You should feel the burn all
the way down the inner thigh to the
knee.)

These two movements (3 and 4) are
done to one count. Repeat for a total
of 20 counts.

Breathing: Exhale as knees come together.

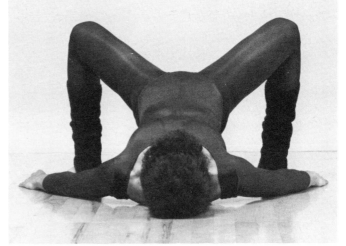

4. Open your knees out again as you
slightly relax your buttocks muscles.

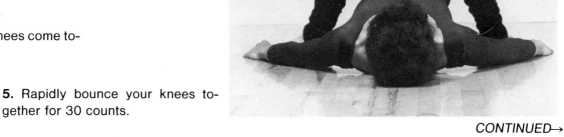

5. Rapidly bounce your knees together for 30 counts.

CONTINUED→

As you bounce the knees together, keep pushing up as hard as you can with your buttocks. Go for the burn! I know it hurts but you'll feel so good afterwards and you'll be so pleased with the results.

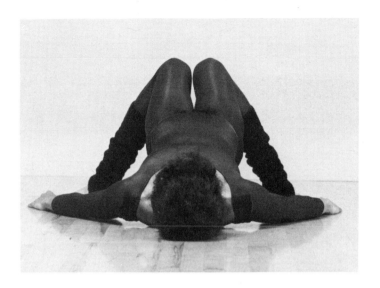

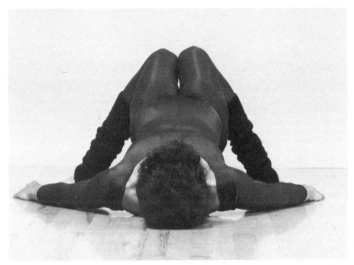

6. Now keep your knees pressed together as you continue to lift and lower your buttocks for 30 counts. Work deep!

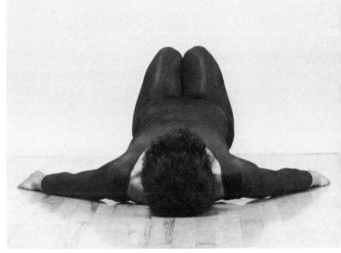

7. Now place your ankles and your knees together and lift the final 20 counts. Whew!

This lifting movement should be very small. What counts is the intensity. You have to work deep. If it burns too much, stop for a brief moment and start again.

If your back aches during this series, it means you are arching it. In this case, concentrate on rounding your lower back as you lift your buttocks.

Breathing: Exhale as you lift, inhale as you lower.

TWO

HIP RELEASE AND STRETCH
Stretches hamstrings and gluteus maximus

1. Extend your left leg out on the floor with the toe pointed. Grab your right foot with both hands and pull the foot across your body, stretching your right hip. This should feel good after what you've just done. Pull gently for 4 counts.

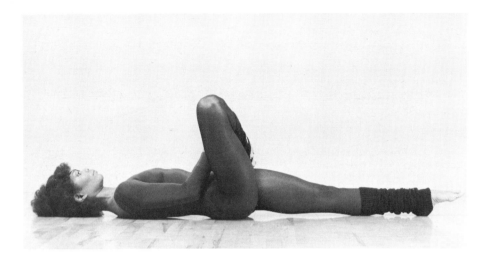

2. Extend your right leg up toward your head, straightening the knee, and pull it toward you with both hands for 4 counts.

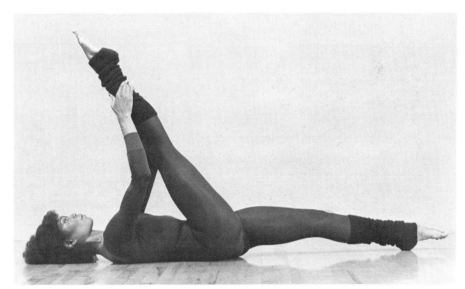

3. Point and flex your foot twice as you pull your leg in to your body.

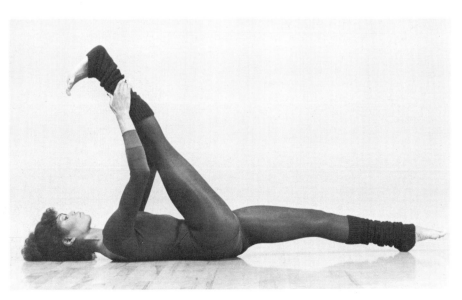

CONTINUED→

4. Change legs, extending your right leg out on the floor while grabbing your left foot with both hands and pulling it across your body for 4 counts.

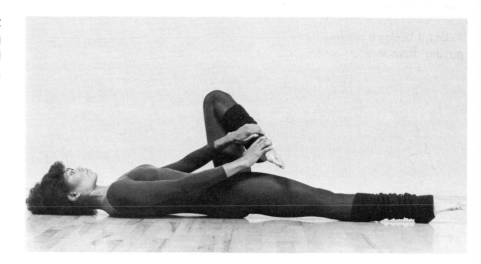

5. Extend your left leg up toward your head and pull it toward you with both hands for 4 counts.

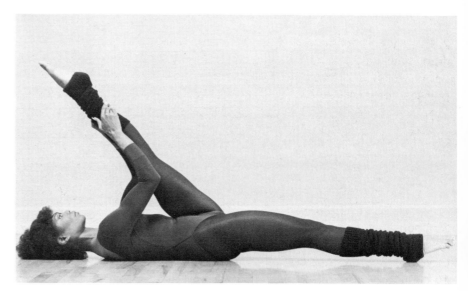

6. Point and flex your left foot twice as you pull your leg into your body.

Breathing: Normal

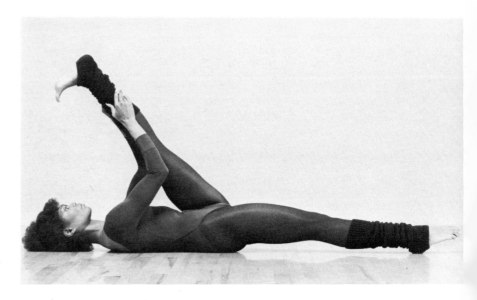

Three HIP AND THIGH RELEASE
Releases inner thigh

1. Bend both knees in to your torso, pulling them in with your hands.

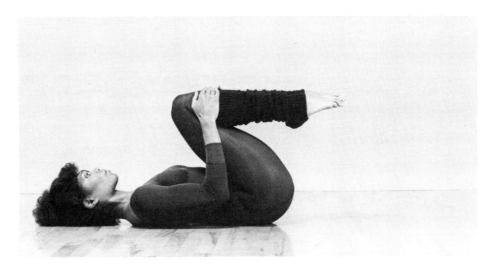

2. Open your knees out to the side, grab both lower legs and press down, releasing slightly between presses, for 8 counts.

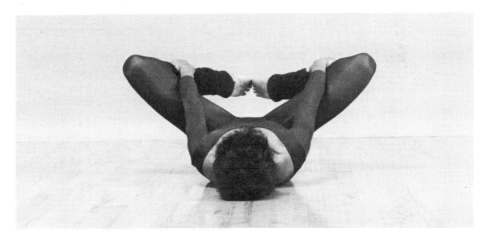

3. Open your legs wide out to the sides, hold on to your ankles or calves and gently bounce down for 16 counts.

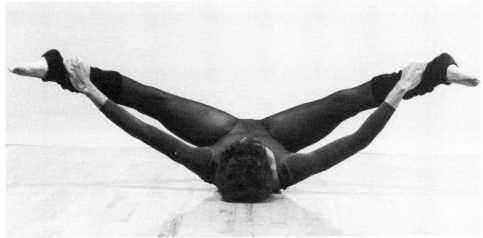

Breathing: Normal

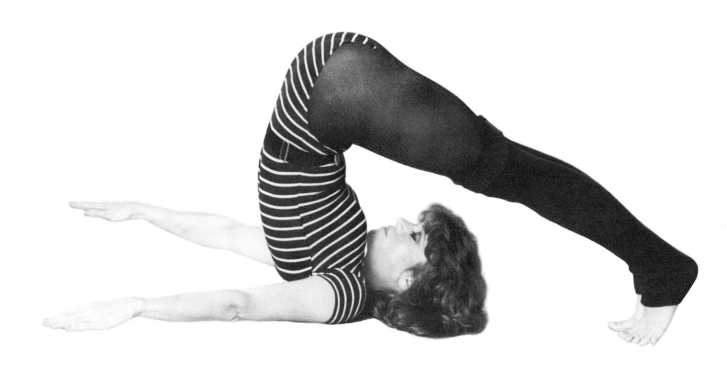

Advanced
COOL-DOWN

COOL-DOWN 3 MINUTES

Purpose: To allow your pulse rate to return to normal and to finish your workout with some excellent yoga stretches.

Music:
Karla Bonoff—"Falling Star" / *Bonoff, Karla*
Karla Bonoff—"Roses in the Garden" / *Bonoff, Karla*
Boz Scaggs—"Harbor Lights" / *Silk Degrees*
Judy Collins—"Houses" / *Judith*
Dan Fogelberg—"Souvenirs" / *Souvenirs*
Jean-François Paillard Chamber Orchestra—"Canon in D" / *Pachelbel—Canon in D*

One   THE FROG

Starting position: Lie on your back, bend your knees outward, press the soles of your feet together and lower your thighs to the floor.

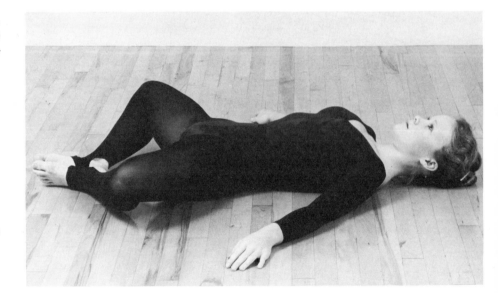

Relax the inner thighs and press the small of the back into the floor.

Breathing: Deep breathing

Two

THE PLOUGH

1. Pull your knees in to your chest.

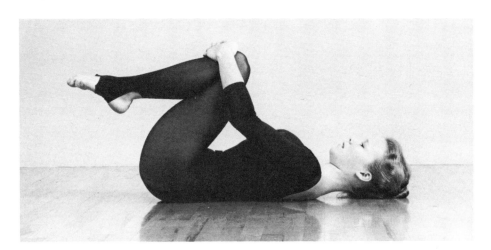

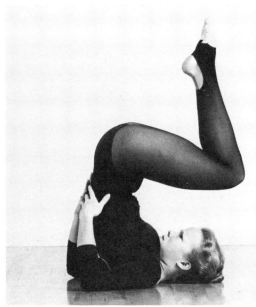

2. Lift your hips up, supporting your lower back with your hands. Bend your knees over your head.

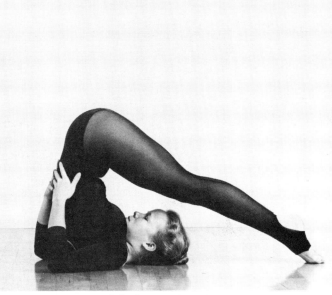

3. Extend your straight legs out past your head as far as you can with pointed toes. Support your lower back with your hands. Hold this position a minute or two if you can.

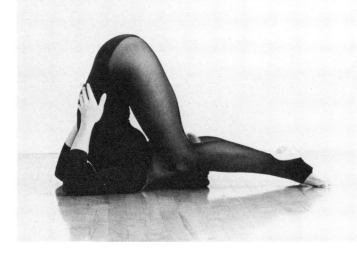

4. Drop your knees toward your ears and hold for a minute.

CONTINUED→

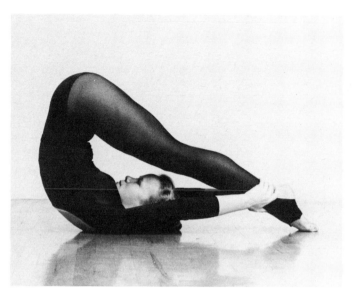

5. Extend your legs out again and grab your ankles with both hands.

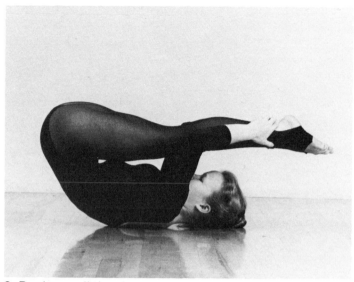

6. Begin to roll down one vertebra at a time. Control the speed at which you roll down by holding your ankles and dragging your legs across your face.

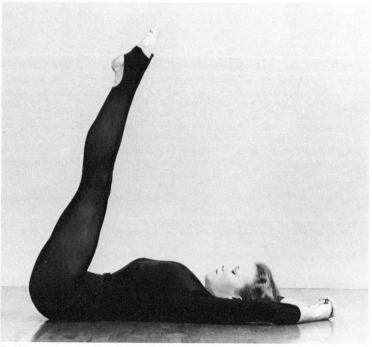

7. When the small of your back is on the floor, let go of your legs.

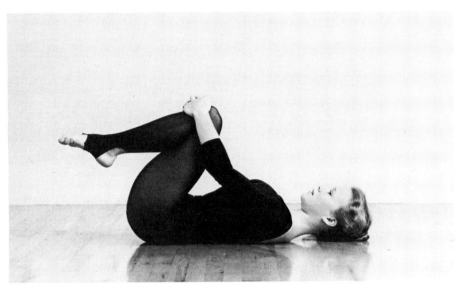

8. Grab your knees and hug them tightly to your chest.

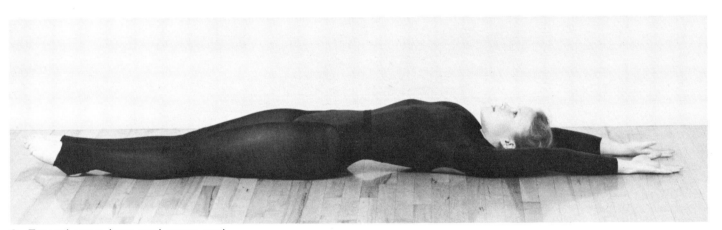

9. Extend your legs and arms and stretch out as far as you can, legs in one direction, arms in the other.

Breathing: Normal

The yoga Plough position is one of the best stretches you can do. It stretches out the spine, allows the vital energy flow to be opened up and, because the chin is being pressed into the chest, stimulates the thyroid gland at the base of the neck. This is the gland that regulates your metabolism.

This is a good position to take when you're tired. If you hold it for 2 minutes and come down very very slowly, you will feel refreshed.

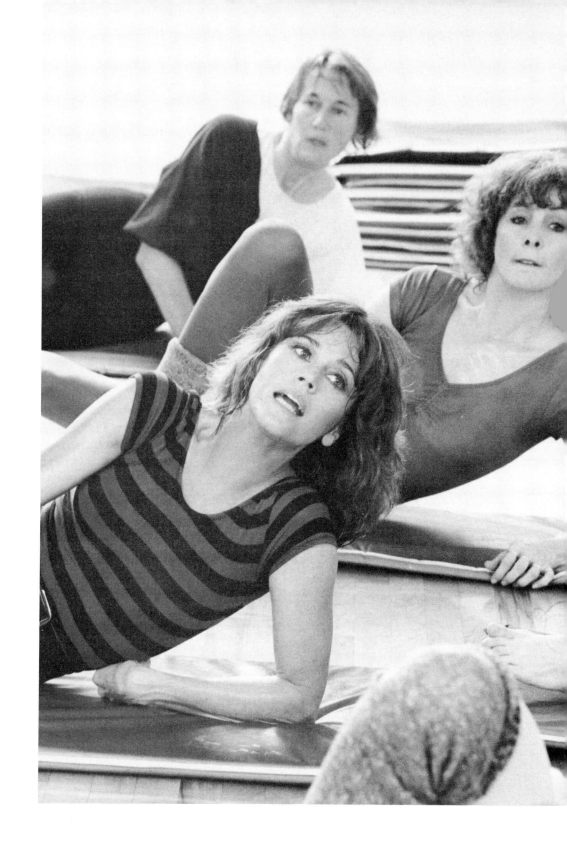

Special Problems

BACKS

Frequently women begin to suffer lower back problems following childbirth. Sometimes the back or pelvis can be thrown out during delivery. Perhaps a visit to a good chiropractor following birth would be good preventive medicine.

Some key things to remember if you suffer pains in your back are:

1. Stand up tall, pulling up out of your torso. Pull your head up but don't stick your chin out.

2. Pull in your lower abdominal muscles and tuck under your pelvis, while elongating and lifting your stomach.

3. Don't stand in one position too long without moving.

4. Avoid wearing high heels all the time, as they shorten the achilles tendon.

5. When sitting, your knees should be higher than your hips when your feet are flat on the ground. The back of the chair should be firm, giving flat support through the upper lumbar region.

6. Never use a chair which sticks into the small of your back.

7. When sitting, short people should put a low stool under their feet if their knees drop below their hips or dangle in the air.

8. Sleep in a firm bed. If your bed is soft, put a ¾″ plywood board under the mattress. A thinner board won't be solid enough.

For those with more serious back problems, here are some special exercises:

One

Starting position: Lie on back with knees bent and feet placed comfortably on the floor, arms over the head.

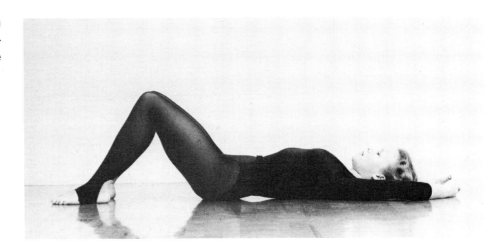

1. Slowly press the small of the back into the floor, slightly tilting the pelvis upward. Exhale as you press the back to the floor. Hold position for 4 counts, then release. Do 3 times.

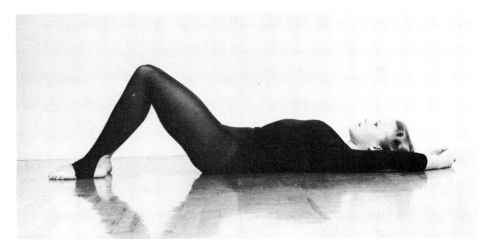

2. Once more, press the small of the back into the floor, then slowly slide the legs out on the floor, trying to keep the small of the back still pressed to the floor.

This action releases tension in the lumbar region or lower back.

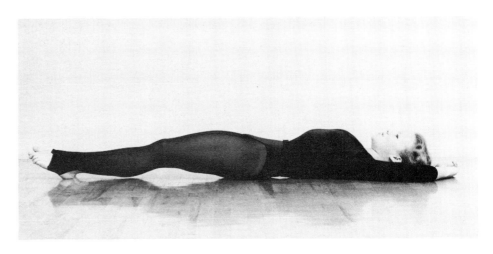

Two

Starting position: Lie on back with knees bent, arms at sides.

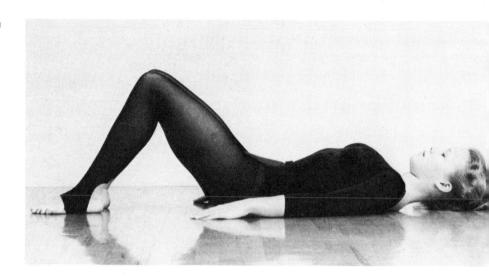

1. Slowly roll up, vertebra by vertebra, keeping chin to chest . . .

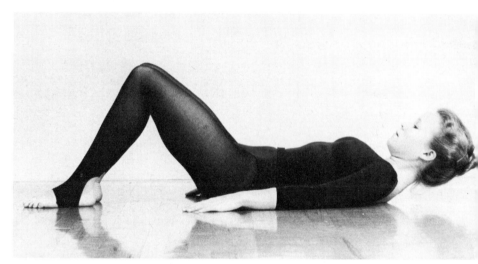

2. . . . until upper back leaves the floor. Exhale as you roll up. Release back to the floor.

Do 5 times. Strengthens abdominals, thereby relieving strain on back.

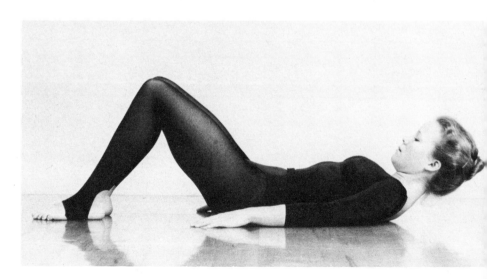

Three

Starting position: Get onto your hands and knees, with knees approximately hip distance apart.

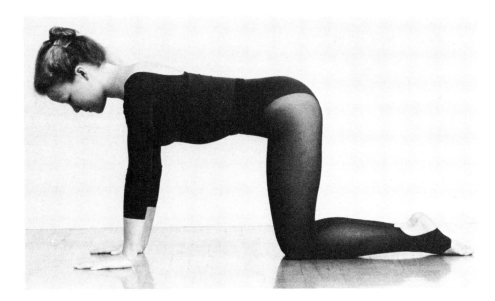

1. Slowly round the back beginning with the lower spine . . .

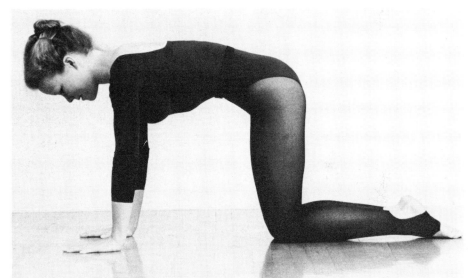

. . . and keeping chin tucked in to chest. Inhale as you round.

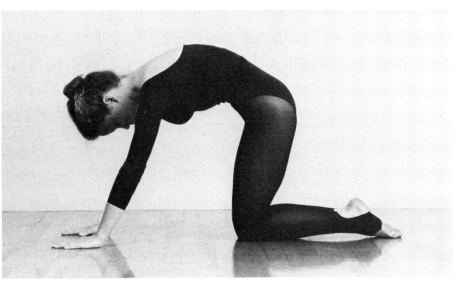

CONTINUED→

2. Release position by relaxing,

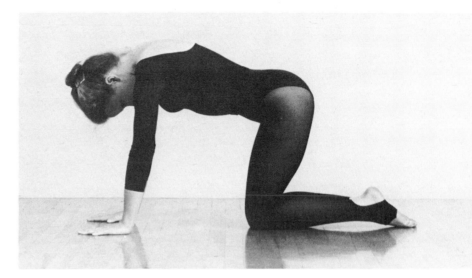

. . . then arch the back beginning with the lower spine . . .

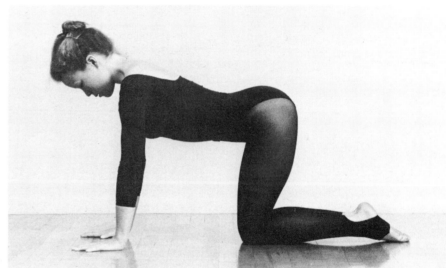

. . . until you lift the head. Exhale as you arch.

Do 5 times. Releases tension in the lumbar region and strengthens lower back.

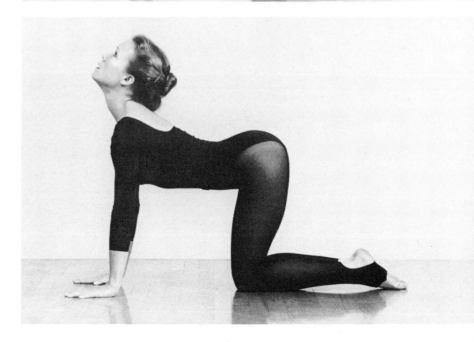

Four

Starting position: Sit in chair, feet flat on floor, legs opened hip distance apart.

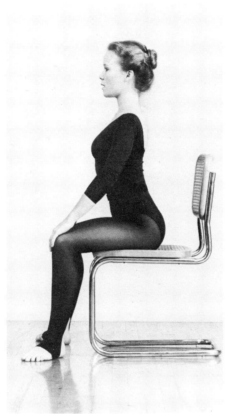

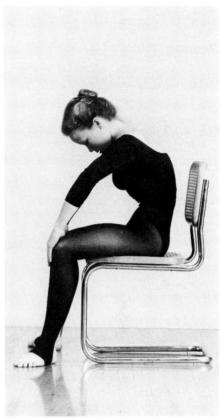

1. Press lower back forward and upward trying to lengthen the spine and lift the chest to the ceiling. Exhale as you press.

2. Release by relaxing.

Do 5 times. Strengthens lower and upper back, lengthens and strengthens particularly the muscles along the spine and loosens the lumbar region for increased flexibility.

Five

Starting position: Stand away from a chair with feet a little more than hip distance apart.

1. Bending forward from the hips, reach out and place hands on the back of the chair, allowing the back to flatten, parallel to the floor.

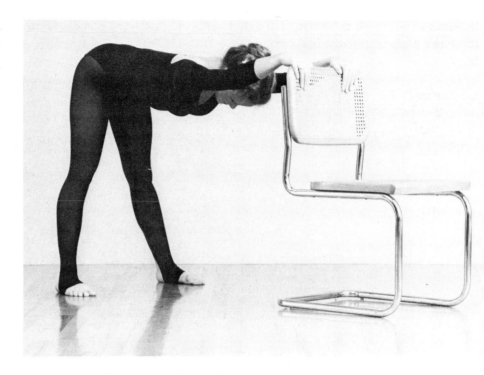

2. Without moving hips, gradually twist torso from the lower back up the spine to your head until you are looking at your right arm. Exhale as you twist.

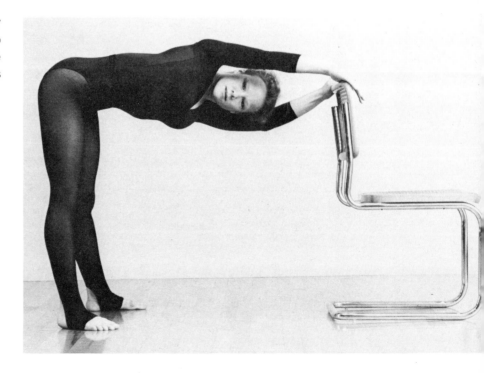

3. Reverse the twist, beginning with the head and ending with the lower back.

Do 2 times to the right, 2 times to the left. Strengthens muscles along spine, particularly those in the lower back.

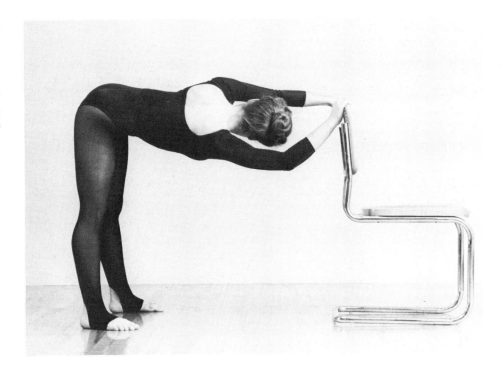

CALVES AND ANKLES

There are many exercises for calves and ankles in the general exercise program. However, for those who want to work further on shaping and toning these areas, here are three of the best exercises:

One

1. Hold on to a chair, table, railing. Stand with your legs wide apart, feet turned out. The wider the stance, the more you'll get out of the movement. Bend your knees so that your buttocks are a little higher than your knees.

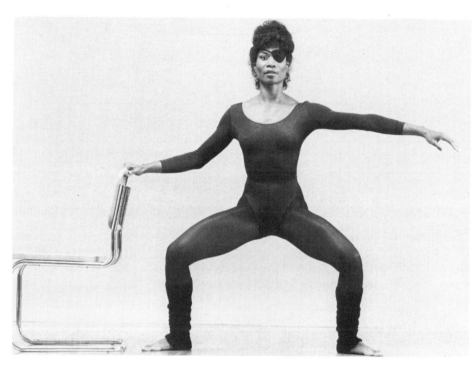

2. Raise your heels as high as you can lift them, then lower them to the floor. When doing this, don't rush and don't move your hips, only your heels. Do it till you can't stand the pain. Do three more, then stop! Shake your legs out and do it again. Keep trying to increase the number you do.

Breathing: Exhale as your raise your heels; inhale as you lower your heels.

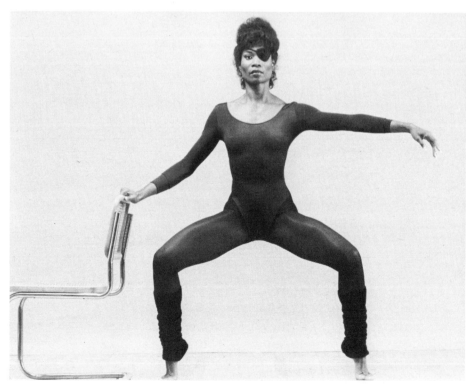

Two

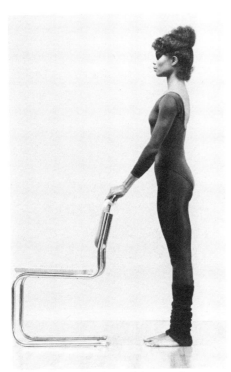

1. Face a chair, table, wall—anything to help you balance. Place your feet parallel to each other, about 6 inches apart.

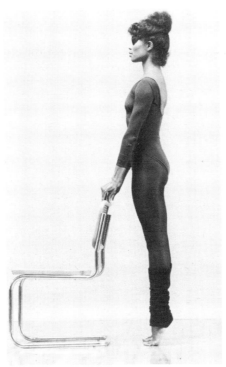

2. Holding lightly on to your support, rise up very high on your toes keeping your stomach flat, buttocks tight, back straight.

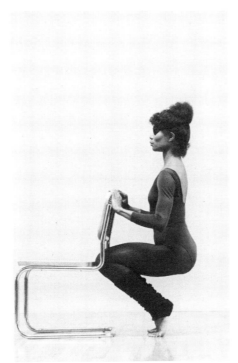

3. Bend your knees and lower your body as far as you can, staying high on your toes.

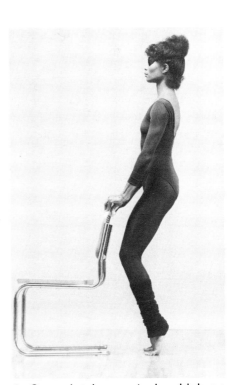

4. Come back up, staying high on your toes. Let your ankles, calves and thighs do the work. Don't pull yourself up with your support.

CONTINUED→

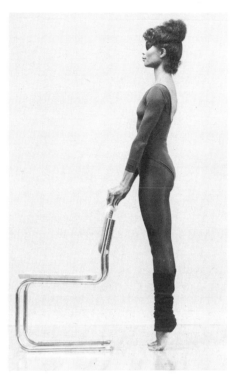 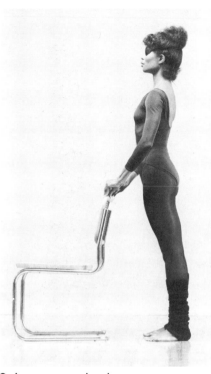

Repeat all 6 movements until you can't lift up anymore. Keep trying to increase the number you do.

Breathing: Normal

5. Come all the way up as high as you can on your toes.

6. Lower your heels.

Three

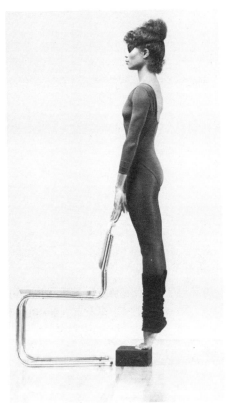

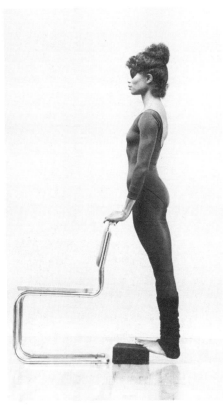

1. Stand on your toes at the edge of a step or block of wood, holding on to something for support.

2. Let your heels drop down as far as they will go below the edge.

3. Rise up again on tiptoe.

Repeat as many times as you are able. If this exercise is too easy, do it with weights on your ankles.

Breathing: Exhale as heels drop down, inhale as you rise.

MENSTRUAL PROBLEMS

Many women experience acute physical and psychological problems before and during the menstrual cycle. Beyond the more common headaches and bloating, symptoms can resemble the wildly fluctuating emotions some of us experience during early pregnancy: irritability, hypersensitivity, depression, fatigue and even compulsive desires for certain foods.

It is now believed these problems are directly related to fluid retention and the ensuing swelling of tissues in the brain as well as the rest of the body.

During this period, two hormones are released which affect salt and fluid retention: aldosterone from the adrenal gland and progesterone from the ovaries.

Exercise is extremely helpful for these problems because, among other things, you sweat more and so lower the amount of fluid and salt in the body.

Several shot-glasses of freshly squeezed parsley juice, a mild diuretic, can help. So can pyridoxine (vitamin B_6), which acts as a diuretic when taken in large doses: 50 to 200 mg.

If your symptoms are more severe, ask your doctor about Aldactone, a mild chemical diuretic that works to suppress the release of the aldosterone hormone. Take these *only during the menstrual cycle.* Even mild, natural diuretics strain the kidneys. The less frequently you take them, the more effect they'll have when you do.

And please don't forget to augment your intake of potassium while using any diuretic. Bananas, dried apricots and tomato juice are good sources of potassium, or you can take potassium chloride if a more concentrated dose is needed.

Generally speaking, the entire exercise program helps alleviate menstrual cramps. For those with continuing problems, here are a few additional movements.

One

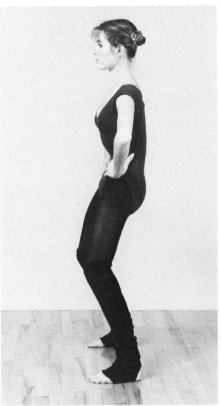

1. Standing with knees slightly bent and feet a little more than hip distance apart, tuck under . . .

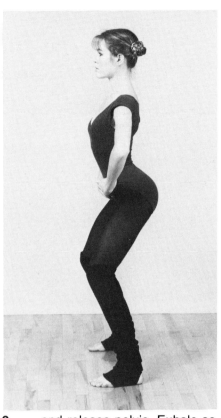

2. . . . and release pelvis. Exhale as you tuck, inhale as you release. Do for 20 counts.

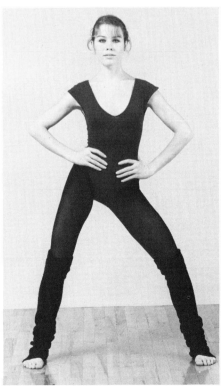

3. Circle pelvis to right for 5 rotations.

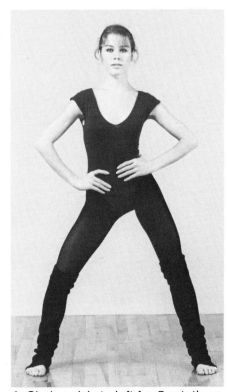

4. Circle pelvis to left for 5 rotations.

TWO

1. With feet a little more than hip distance apart, lower into a "squatting" position making sure knees are bent directly over toes and heels remain on the floor. Allow hips to relax downward toward floor and gently sway from side . . .

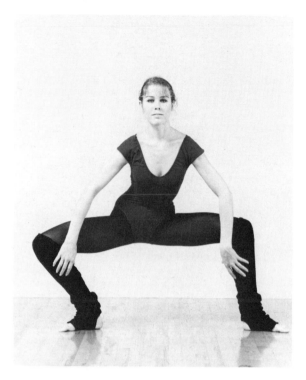

2. . . . to side. Steady breathing. Do for 10 counts.

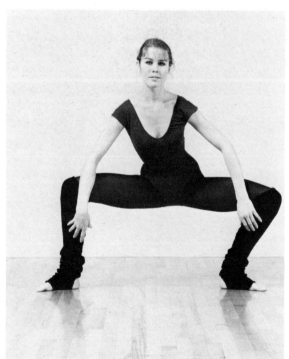

Three

1. Lying flat on back with knees bent and feet comfortably on floor, inhale and pull abdominals in and hold for 5 counts.

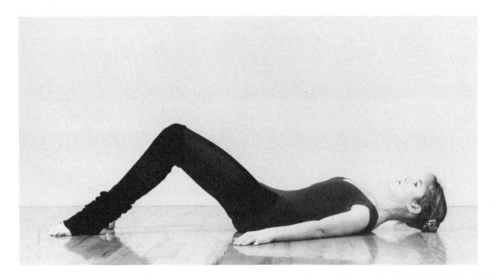

2. Exhale and release abdominals for 5 counts.

Pull in and release 10 times.

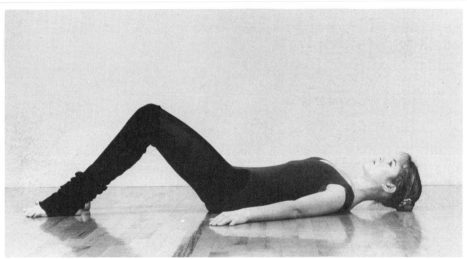

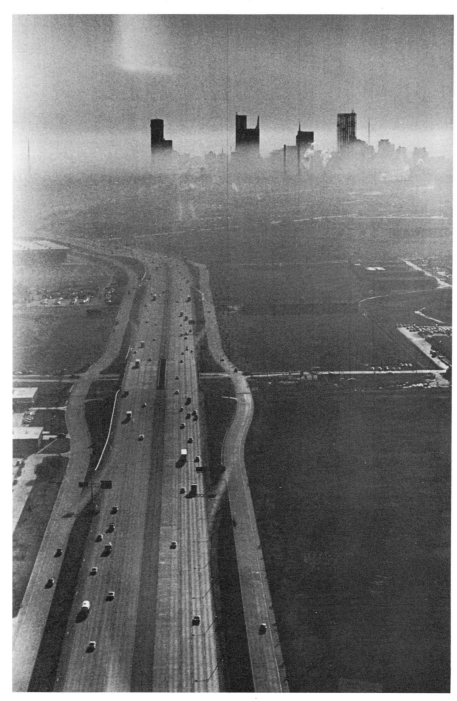

Part Five
The Body Besieged

When you read the following section, I know that some of you will say "There she goes! Fonda can't just tell us to eat properly and exercise regularly and leave it at that. She wants to change the world."

Well, in some ways I do. Everyone knows I'm an activist. There is no way I can write about health and leave it at urging you to make a personal commitment to nutrition and exercise. I am truly heartened by the fact that in increasing numbers we are making a more aggressive commitment to health, to regular exercise and to eating more nutritious meals; but the fact is that we can only be as healthy as our ecological environment—the one true life-support system. If that is out of whack, then our individual life-style decisions are mere righteous gestures. We must become aware of how we are being affected by our environment and what actions we can take to protect ourselves, as individuals, as communities, and as part of the whole ecosystem.

After you read these chapters, you may want to add a little activism to your own approach to health. I hope so. If you do, you will find some suggestions for getting started at the end of the book.

Retreat from Victory

Not so very long ago when my parents were growing up, people lived in a world where health seemed the inevitable result of progress:

Tuberculosis was no longer a dread major killer, now that modern sanitation and progressive housing codes were correcting the terrible living conditions in city tenements.

Thanks to rigorous mosquito control, malaria and yellow fever—which were once endemic, particularly in the South—had been practically wiped out.

The quality of drinking water was now being monitored, with the result that cholera and other water-borne diseases were no longer a threat.

And milk was safe to drink. Pasteurization, then the only technologically feasible way to provide safe milk for a large population, had been bitterly opposed by the dairy industry. We have the efforts of women's organizations to thank for winning the fight for pasteurization.

Clean, unadulterated food and drugs were being guaranteed by federal inspection, in response to the public's indignation over scandals exposed in newspapers, magazines and such novels as Upton Sinclair's *The Jungle.*

Disease and death in the workplace were beginning to come under close scrutiny as major industries became unionized. Through these unions, workers were claiming more of a say about their working conditions—not only with regard to hours and wages, but about health hazards like lead poisoning and exposure to metal dusts and other toxic by-products of the manufacturing process. By the 1940s, Dr. Alice Hamilton, the founder of occupational medicine in this country and the first woman ever appointed to the faculty of Harvard University, was able to reflect in her autobiography that the control of hazards on the job was a goal that might soon be achieved.

Children may have benefited most from these advances that took place during my parents' youth and continued through my childhood. Infant mortality, one of the most sensitive measures of overall health, diminished significantly. Inoculation to prevent and, later on, antibiotics to cure were eliminating the infectious diseases that had been the major

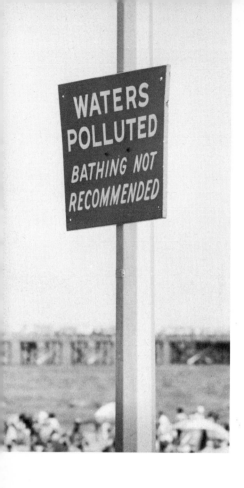

killers of children. Even dread polio was finally conquered, and it was safe to go in the water again. Or so we thought.

Given all these victories, one might think that a sensible personal life style was all that was needed to ensure relatively good health. The air was clean in those days. People's routines at work and at home were less sedentary. Food came from your garden, or from a grocery store that got it straight from a local farm.

A little common sense was all that was needed. Or so it seemed. That old adage, "An apple a day keeps the doctor away," must have been born of such optimism. Nowadays, however, such a laissez-faire attitude toward health isn't good enough. Too many detrimental external factors are besieging us in the food we eat, on the job where we work and in our environment: before you eat that apple, you'd better check to see what it's been sprayed with.

When I was a child in Los Angeles, there was rarely a day when we couldn't see across the basin from the San Gabriel Mountains out to Catalina Island in the distance. I spent my summers playing in the surf at Santa Monica Beach. My daughter Vanessa, however, did not know for years that Los Angeles was ringed by mountains, because she couldn't see them. We live a block and a half from the beach at Santa Monica now, yet Vanessa is reluctant to go swimming there.

She is afraid of getting cancer, and she has reason to be afraid. Five lifeguards who worked on the beach contracted cancer. It is suspected that their disease is linked to toxic chemicals that had been dumped into a sewage drain that spills out onto the beach near the lifeguard station, where its contents then flow into the ocean less than a mile from where I played as a child.

People in Santa Monica think twice these days before turning on the faucet for a glass of water. Many of us drink bottled water instead. Not too long ago one of the city's main wells was temporarily closed when it was found to be contaminated with trichloroethylene (a cancer-causing chemical). The well had been sunk right through an abandoned chemical waste dump which was leaching chemicals into the water.

It is little comfort to us in Santa Monica to know that we are not alone and that hundreds of municipal wells from Southern California to Tennessee to Long Island have been similarly contaminated. In 1980, a Congressional committee examining this subject concluded, "The health of millions of Americans is threatened by government and industry's past failure to properly protect our groundwater."

Here in Los Angeles, we get used to a certain amount of smog, especially during the summer, but in October 1980, the smog was so heavy that children were throwing up at school. My son, Troy, who was seven at the time, was one of them. His eyes were sunken and red-rimmed and he felt nauseated, tired and irritable for weeks. A woman who lives in nearby San Fernando Valley told me that her little boy had passed out in school.

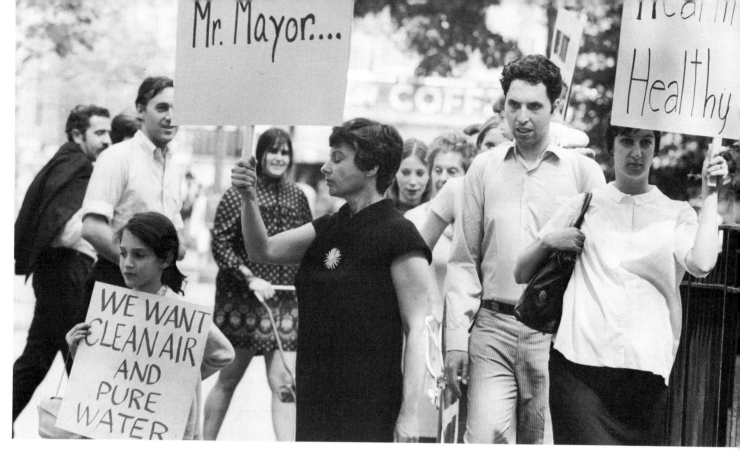

I developed a rash on my face and a throat infection that took weeks to clear up. Many of my friends had the same symptoms. Hospitals in the Los Angeles area reported a heavy overload of respiratory victims. Even more frightening was the way people's behavior changed. We became irritable, snapping at each other. Some people found it was becoming difficult to think clearly. I felt as if my brain were stuffed with cotton.

In the middle of this crisis, Ronald Reagan, then campaigning for the Presidency, was quoted as saying that he felt air pollution was under ''substantial control.'' Must our children sicken and die like canaries in a mine shaft before he recognizes that pollution remains a serious question? My question is valid in view of the fact that his administration has delayed even further the enforcement of auto emission standards that would help clean up the air.

One of the reasons Tom and I moved to Santa Monica was to escape the smog. We moved, but we did not escape. Here we are living in a nice middle-class community, perched next to the ocean on the western edge of our continent in this sunny city that has beckoned to utopia seekers for almost a century—and we are afraid to swim in the ocean, sick from breathing the air and unable to drink the water.

If anyone had told me fifteen years ago that I would tolerate living under these conditions, I would have thought he was not playing with a full deck. Yet here we are. Our work, our children's school, our home, our commitments all keep us here. We know that we could move again, go someplace else, but we also know that eventually you run out of mountaintops to escape to. We can't run away. We have to stay like so many others, and like them, we have to figure out what to do about it.

What has happened to the victories that were won by my grandparents' and parents' generations, to be safeguarded by us for our own children? Infant mortality, which had been on the decline, has now leveled off—far above the rate of other industrialized countries. Our water, which had been cleansed of cholera, is now contaminated with chemical discharges more insidious, if less immediately deadly. Our air, free from the threat of disease-carrying mosquitoes, now carries the sting of petrochemical pollutants. Our food supply is more adulterated than ever before. And the workplace, far from being under control, is a testing ground where millions of working women and men are exposed daily to new chemicals and processes whose long-range health effects have never been ascertained.

The food we eat, the air we breathe, the water we drink, the contaminants present in our workplaces—contaminants that are inhaled or absorbed through the skin—all bear directly on our health. All our life-support systems have undergone a major transformation within the last three decades that is going to have ever-increasing and disastrous effects on our national well-being if allowed to continue.

As women we can have a lot to say about this. We are the ones after all who buy and prepare the food. We are the ones who can influence our children's eating habits instead of leaving it up to television. The quality of the environment that our children will inherit is being determined now. We musn't surrender that responsibility to corporate interests. More of us are part of the work force than ever before, and we cannot afford to pay the price of a workplace environment that is unhealthy and stressful. It will be up to us to win safe and humane living conditions.

Let's start by taking a look at what's happened to the American dinner.

Overfed and Undernourished

I love to eavesdrop when I'm standing in lines, especially lines of people waiting for food. Recently, I overheard this conversation at Magic Mountain among a group of teenagers, all of them with bad complexions. One girl was ordering a chocolate milkshake. Her friends admonished her to get some *real* food. "You haven't had anything to eat for twenty-four hours," one said. "You've got to have something better than a milkshake."

"Okay," the girl said. And added a bag of french fries to her order.

"That's better," another one of her friends approved. "And tonight we'll go to Taco Bell for a *real* dinner."

Fast food has become the real dinner for too many of us. Kids are growing up never knowing the taste of a sun-ripened tomato. Some youngsters believe that chickens have six legs because that's how many legs there are in a package. And how many mothers think Tang is orange juice? That "crispy" is a taste? And that nutrition is synthetic vitamins sprayed on the "Breakfast of Champions"? Will 1984's answer to "How was dinner, darling?" be "Convenient"?

Something has happened to the American dinner and a lot of people are taking it sitting down. Cozy down-home brand names like Mrs. Butterworth's Syrup, Dad's Root Beer and Ma Brown's Ol-Fashun Pickles make us feel there is still a competitive entrepreneurial spirit, alive and well, which is providing us with well-prepared foods from the kitchens of a caring family business. The fact is, however, that the British-Dutch conglomerate Unilever owns the syrup, Illinois Central Railroad owns the root beer, and Beatrice Foods Company, a three-billion-dollar-a-year multi-national conglomerate that manufactures five thousand food items, brings us Ma Brown's pickles. ITT, Procter and Gamble, United Brands and General Foods are among the fifty companies that reap about 70 percent of the total profits of the food industry. The giant conglomerates have gained monopoly control over breakfast, lunch and dinner.

As they gobble up their competition, corraling thousands of brand

APPETIZERS

Sautéed Mushrooms by Clorox wrapped in
Bacon by ITT
Salmon by Unilever

SALADS

Tossed Salad of Lettuce by Dow Chemical
and Tomatoes by Gulf & Western
Avocado Salad by Superior Oil

ENTREES

Turkey by Ling-Temco-Vought
Ham by Greyhound
Roast Beef by Oppenheimer Industries

SIDE DISHES

Artichokes by Purex
Carrots by Tenneco
Potatoes by Boeing
Apple Sauce by American Brands
Deviled Eggs by Cargill
Olives by Zapata Oil

BEVERAGE

Wine by Heublein
Citrus Juice by Pacific Lighting Corp.

AFTER DINNER

Peaches by Westgate-California Corp.
Almonds by Getty Oil

233

names into their corporate stable, some of the companies extend their control vertically as well. They buy, for instance, the seed and fertilizer companies and sometimes the land the food is grown on, the means of transporting the food and the packaging and processing companies. Frequently they have their own food outlets, which may include public restaurants, vending machines and food-service concessions with airlines, hotels, hospitals, and so on.

A small entrepreneur might come up with a fantastically delicious and extremely nutritious breakfast cereal, but she or he would have practically no chance against the big boys with their lock on the marketplace and their tens of millions of advertising dollars.

"Anyone who likes what Detroit's Big Three have done for automobiles," Jim Hightower has written in his book *Eat Your Heart Out*, "will be pleased with these emerging food systems, for the same quality, price competition, choice and product reliability are being built into the food we eat." Well, there is hope here. Americans voted against Detroit's automobiles with their pocketbooks in 1980 and 1981. We can vote the same way against over-processed foods by insisting on more natural foods and fewer additives, by eating lower on the food chain and eating more fresh foods. But it won't be easy. Just try to get your Big Mac on a whole wheat bun or low-fat yogurt from your local vending machine. Try, for that matter, to get fresh fruit or skim milk on an airplane. Nutritious food is hard to come by.

CONCENTRATION MEANS INFLATION

If you are concerned about the rise in the cost of food, you have the monopolies to thank. The giants get away with inflated prices because there is so little competition and we have nowhere else to go—or think we don't. We paid at least $16 billion too much for the food we bought in 1980, according to a Department of Agriculture estimate, because of the stranglehold of the monopolies. This amounted to nearly 6 percent of the average amount spent on food per household.

Advertising is one of the main costs passed along to the consumer. Three billion dollars is spent on food advertising every year and 90 percent of that is for television. Commercials for snack foods, candy bars and sugary breakfast cereals are the mainstay of children's TV programs. Commercials for processed and packaged foods get prime air time, while fresh vegetables, yeast and whole grain bread have no sponsors.

Food is displayed in supermarkets to emphasize sugary and processed items. Have you ever noticed how processed foods are always in the "end of aisle" displays which are the key sales areas? And sweets are most often displayed at a child's-eye level. Economical and nutritious foods like beans and brown rice are rarely featured, because their low prices are not conducive to billion-dollar profits. Convenience foods are promoted because they are more profitable. The less natural a food product is, the more it has been tampered with, the more they can charge for it.

Take two ordinary baking potatoes. As I write this, they cost 69 cents at my supermarket. If those potatoes are peeled and canned, the price goes up by a dime. If they are processed into potato chips, a pound will increase to $1.19 and your weight will increase as well. By weight, potato chips have six times as many calories, 250 times as much salt and 400 times as much fat as a baked potato.

Processing and packaging make food look fancier but, what is more important, they enable it to stay on the shelf almost indefinitely without spoiling. The processing and packing make it easy to ship food around the world, thus gaining a vastly enlarged marketplace for the product. Never mind that you and I end up paying more for the processing and packaging than we do for the food itself, or that American meals are turning into servings of neutered convenience foods and adulterated snacks in fast-food chains. That is where the profits lie and that is what it has come down to.

The corporate response to the mounting public concern about health and nutrition has not been to use a portion of their profits to improve the quality of their food. They continue to remove many of the essential vitamins, minerals and dietary fibers during the processing, then to "fortify" the product by adding a few synthetic nutrients, and spend huge sums selling the product as "enriched and nutritious" at enriched prices.

General Mills, the conglomerate that brings us Wheaties, The Breakfast of Champions, is an example. We are sold Wheaties for $1.21, although there is only two cents' worth of wheat in Wheaties. The box costs more than the wheat. Writer Jim Hightower suggests that we would be getting about the same nutritional value if we tore up the box, added milk and ate it.

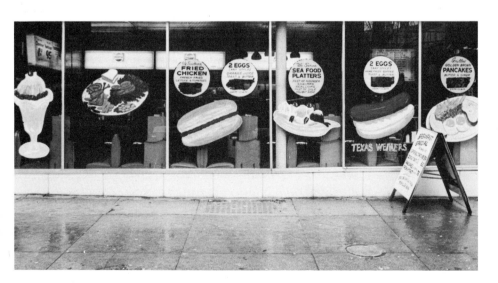

In response to consumer interest in nutrition, General Mills came out with a new cereal, Total. Total is nothing but Wheaties with an extra two cents' worth of synthetic vitamins sprayed on. Though it costs General Mills about two cents more to produce a 12-ounce box of Total, the consumer pays up to 42 cents more for it! Outrageous, you say? Yes, it is. But with a multi-million dollar advertising budget, they actually persuade us to buy this stuff at that price. They have made millions of dollars on just this one scheme.

With television as the arbiter of what's best to eat, we are swapping taste for speed, the genuine for the synthetic, health for convenience. The marketing of these manufactured foods swells the profits of the big conglomerates, but it is taking a serious toll on our nation's health. A majority of the essential vitamins, minerals and trace elements that are necessary for good health are removed by milling, refining, flaking, puffing and shredding. And only a very few of these essentials are replaced by "enriching."

While looking for lost nutrients in the never-never land of corporate cookery, you're more likely to discover a host of truly exotic substances whose names will not exactly flow trippingly from the tongue (unless you're a biochemist).

Imagine if some fast-food chain had to put a complete list of ingredients on the menu and you had to order them by full name. You might starve to death before getting "butylated hydroxytoluene," "heptyl-hydroxydenzoate," and "sodium propionate" communicated to the server. But that's what the "new meal" is about these days.

There are about 2500 substances added to our food. According to Jim Hightower, the average American eats 6.7 pounds of food additives per year. "Hundreds of these chemicals have not been tested enough to know with any certainty that they are safe to eat, nor is there any real knowledge as to how these 2500 ingredients react to each other when they come together in the stomach."

An article in Fortune that supported the use of additives nonetheless acknowledged that there was some reason for concern, saying that "there have been some alarming discoveries over recent years suggesting that quite a few substances can react with, and thereby alter, the composition of the DNA molecules that make up the vital genetic blueprints for all living species."

Food additives are dangerous not only as mutagens and carcinogens. Many, including the widely used yellow dye No. 5, cause allergic reactions in some people, upset the delicate balances within the body and impede the absorption of essential vitamins and minerals. Hyperactivity and learning disabilities in some children have been linked to food colorings and flavorings.

If it's true, as some say, that you are what you eat, some of us might have more in common with a chemist's test tube than with our great grandmothers.

Instead of blindly giving in to the food conglomerates' influences, like dietary lemmings, many citizens' groups, women's organizations and PTAs have fought back. As a result of their efforts, advertising on children's TV programs has been reduced from 16 minutes to 9 minutes per hour. More public service announcements focus on proper eating habits. School lunch programs have been made more nutritional (although now we must fight to retain them altogether). There are more food co-ops, farmers' markets and urban gardens because citizens' groups have organized to eliminate the food processors and food middlemen and get food straight from the farmer to the community. Farm workers—women, men, and children together—have organized under leaders such as Cesar Chávez to demand controls on pesticides that poison them in the fields and consumers down the food chain. Agricultural alternatives to petrochemical poisons being sprayed indiscriminately—such as Integrated Pest Management—are gaining ground. In 1967, when I first became interested in nutrition, the Adelle Davis books were the only place to turn for advice on eating for health. Now, even Dr. Julius B. Richmond, the former Surgeon General, has advised us that we should eat whole wheat bread. This symbolizes a great step forward in legitimizing the nutritional point of view and it is the result of public demands.

As these examples show, it *is* possible to make a difference. We Americans, who pride ourselves on our individuality and claim to cherish our freedom of choice, must not give up our right to control something as fundamental as what we put into our bodies. "If anything ought to be real in our lives, ought to be left to nature rather than being simulated by corporate technicians, it is food," Jim Hightower says. "Monopolistic conglomerates cannot make our telephones work; why should they be arrogant enough to think that they can handle dinner? More to the point, why should we be dumb enough to let them?"

A good question. Don't you agree?

The Cancer Scandal

Chemicals in our food represent only one of the ways our bodies are being besieged. Few people need convincing these days that we are in the midst of a cancer epidemic. One person dies of cancer every minute and a quarter, according to the American Cancer Society, and one out of every four persons in this country will have cancer. At the turn of the century, it was only one person out of 25, by the turn of this century, it may be every other person.

Cancer has become a major killer in our lifetime, not simply because people have stopped dying of other causes: even when all other factors are taken into account, the absolute incidence of cancer is steadily, but not inevitably, on the rise. This year, it will claim more than 400,000 nationwide. There is hardly anyone who does not have a friend or relative touched by this dreadful disease.

Millions have been spent for research into cures for cancer, but except for a few remarkable advances—childhood leukemia, for example—we seem no closer to a cure than before. Few real gains have been made against the major killers, cancers of the lung, breast, colon, prostate and pancreas.

But suppose the answer lay in an entirely different approach? Suppose we tried to control cancer by *prevention* rather than by cure? It is entirely possible that this is within our ability today. It may have been yesterday, But even though it is widely accepted that much of our cancer can be stopped through prevention, little has been done to make this possibility a reality. De facto economic policies functioning in the name of profit and progress find it cheaper to keep to "business as usual," to spend millions for research into possible cures and nothing to implement prevention.

Why is this happening? We have all grown up surrounded by myths and half-myths about the causes of cancer. Some believe it is hereditary, infectious, caused by physical trauma or weakened resistance. Even "negative vibes" are blamed. But gradually, as the studies come in, we are left staring into the very nature of the society we live in: cancer is a by-product of the petrochemical age.

These reports conclude that virtually all of us in the United States carry in our bodies one or more of the long-lasting synthetic chemicals known to cause severe health problems at higher dosage levels. Commenting on these studies, former Surgeon General Dr. Julius B. Richmond has stated that we are dealing with one of the most serious, and very possibly the worst, threat to human health in the nation today. The World Health Organization reports that 80 percent of all cancer is "environmentally related." This means that we are exposed to carcinogens in the workplace, in the environment, in our food, and as a result of our life styles (such as smoking, and eating a high-fat, low-fiber diet).

The National Cancer Institute estimates that 20 percent of cancer incidence today is at least partially caused by exposure in the workplace. And that figure will zoom up to 40 percent in the years ahead. The Institute predicts that among the population exposed to asbestos, more than two million will die of cancer. This is more than all the men killed in all the wars in our country's history.

Asbestos fibers have been used for more than sixty years as insulation material, and the danger of exposure to these fibers threatens far beyond the factory door. Wives of asbetos workers have contracted cancer from inhaling the dust while washing their husbands' work clothes. Children have gotten seriously ill from playing near asbestos waste. The Environmental Protection Agency estimates that ten thousand schools (around the country) may pose a hazard to children because of asbestos insulation. In my own work, film lighting and technical crews have been unnecessarily exposed to the hazards of asbestos electrical insulation. Millions of American women were exposed to asbestos used in hair dryers.

Asbestos is only one on a very long list of dangerous substances to which people have been carelessly exposed. Since the 1940s an explosion of exotic new chemical products has showered down on us—and most of them have not been tested for carcinogenic effects. Asbestos waste is only a small part of the 57 million tons of hazardous waste produced every year, and according to the EPA up to 90 percent

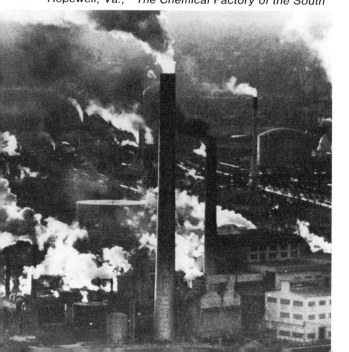

Hopewell, Va., "The Chemical Factory of the South"

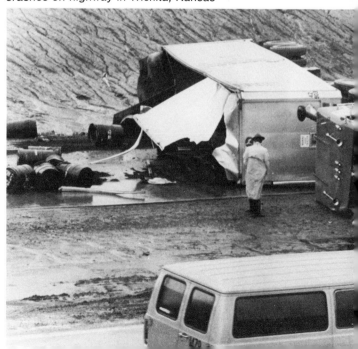

Trailer truck carrying drums of radioactive uranium crashes on highway in Wichita, Kansas

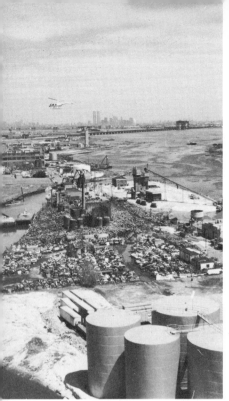
Elizabeth, N.J., waterfront devastated by chemical dump fire

of it is dumped improperly. Public interest lawyer and writer Mark Green calls these dumps "toxic time bombs," of which Love Canal is only the most publicized. The time-bomb metaphor is apt. The average period of latency (which is the time elapsing before a cancer becomes medically evident) following exposure to carcinogens is twenty years or more. The cancer epidemic we are now witnessing is the result of exposures that took place twenty to thirty years ago when the petrochemical industry was in its infancy. Imagine what we are going to face in another couple of decades!

Cancer is not the only damage these toxic chemicals do to our bodies. They have been shown to cause birth defects, neurologic damage, sterility, mental disorders and death from diseases of the blood, kidneys, lungs and other less well known—but no less fatal—diseases than cancer. When the chemical companies say that something they make will touch your life, they are not kidding.

The 1940s also saw a different kind of explosion. Its legacy has been left in weapon stockpiles, in reactor fuel-core piles and in toxic radioactive waste piles. Radioactive waste lies leaking in rusted drums in our oceans, buried in our land—and more waste is being made every day. Scientists admit that there is no answer in sight to the problem of radioactive waste. But plans still go forward for more nuclear power plant licensing and more waste from increased weapons production. These will add to our burden of cancer, birth defects and other diseases.

What can we do? First of all we need to alert ourselves to the dangers we face, but we must not let ourselves be immobilized by them. Cancer is not inevitable. Along with all the other myths about cancer, there is the popular one that "everything causes cancer, so what the hell." This is a dangerous attitude. Science has shown us that some chemicals that are widely used and distributed can and do cause cancer. But science has also shown us that the vast majority of substances are free of such risk. The carcinogens that do exist can be identified, minimized and in many cases, eliminated. It is important to keep two facts in mind:

Everything does not cause cancer.
There are solutions to these problems.

The emphasis of scientific and medical cancer research has been on looking for elusive, costly hi-tech cures. During the 1970s, the budget of the National Cancer Institute—the government's "pentagon" for the War on Cancer—rose to 937 million dollars (almost one billion), but very little of that money went to prevention. It would make sense to allocate our funds to searching out and eliminating the *causes* of disease, the way our parents and their parents did successfully. But this is not happening. In fact, the situation is quite the opposite. It has been proposed to cut the budget of the Center for Disease Control, the main federal institute for disease prevention, by more than 40 percent. The regulatory and enforcement capabilities of such agencies as the Occupational Safety and Health Administration, The Consumer Product Safety Commission and the Environmental Protection Agency are all under attack by the current administration.

Our representatives in Washington must be made aware that the prevention of disease is one of the most reliable weapons in the fight against inflation. A product that causes cancer does not reflect its true costs when we look at its price as it sits on the market shelf. The workers who make it and the consumers who buy it subsidize its production with their health and lives. These costs are incalculable and frightening.

Even Union Carbide, in a public-opinion survey it commissioned in 1979, discovered that 70 percent of the public favor stricter standards than are presently on the books to protect workers from health risks like cancer, and 65 percent favor similar strictness to protect consumers— even though they believe that such controls might raise consumer prices. Washington seems to have forgotten what the rest of us still remember—that an ounce of prevention is worth a pound of cure.

There are specific ways in which state and federal controls can be strengthened. One of the most important is to hold corporations that produce or handle hazardous materials strictly liable for the damage those materials cause. It seems unbelievable, but victims of toxic poisoning usually have to prove that their illness was the result of *deliberate* negligence by a company, not just the result of poor management, ignorance or greed. If companies are not held liable, it is you and I who foot the bill. It is like being forced to subsidize corporate mismanagement.

Another change that must be made is making the "right to know" legal and mandatory in every state. It is neither a federal nor in most cases a state crime for a corporation to suppress information about the adverse effects of its chemical products. In fact, bills that guarantee workers the basic right to know what they are being exposed to on the job have only now begun to be passed in such states as California and New York. They should be introduced in every state.

There is even more that we can do on the local level. A consumer "right to know" law, which gives a community the power to find out what chemicals are in use within its boundaries, has just been enacted for the first time in Philadelphia. Other communities have united to control hazardous cargoes that have traveled unmonitored and unnoticed over their roads and railroads until a disaster has revealed that neither local nor state officials were prepared to handle such hazards.

No single issue has threatened communities more directly than the unsafe disposal of chemical wastes. Seemingly overnight, a quiet, comfortable neighborhood can turn into a hell of oozing chemical sludge, battered hopes and broken health. According to Dr. Samuel Epstein, the cancer expert, there is no such thing as a secure landfill for toxic chemicals. Dr. Epstein believes that by providing permanent landfills for these chemicals, we remove the incentive for finding safer

Love Canal

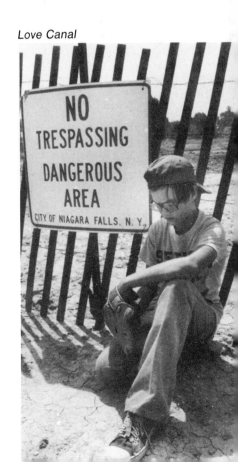

methods for disposal. There are many biological, chemical and physical methods available today for the treatment of much of the chemical waste that is now dumped in the landfills. Dr. Epstein also states that the major expansion of new detoxification strategies (neutralization, solidification, high temperature incineration), as well as recycling waste and changing production techniques to reduce waste at the source, are alternatives to current dumping practices. Such alternatives would protect our health, are economically viable, would stimulate new technology and save energy at the same time. Economic incentives must be created to make these forms of disposal more attractive than dumping.

Chemical waste and contaminated water, air pollution and toxic hazards on the job, cancer, birth defects . . . the list seems endless and the situation overwhelming. Most people just keep on going, hoping they will not become another statistic, an early casualty. In general, they are pessimistic. What can one person do, they ask.

I myself am optimistic, and Lois Gibbs is one reason why. Lois, rather shy and not very social, was a more or less typical housewife and mother of two children. Her time was taken up with caring for her home and family.

What made Lois different was that she lived in Love Canal. Her children's school was built on a toxic chemical dump in that now-famous region of Niagara Falls, New York. As she watched her two youngsters develop serious and inexplicable health problems, she began to realize they were somehow related to the dump. She began a petition drive to get the school closed.

She encouraged her neighbors to talk about the health problems in their own households. They turned out to include multiple miscarriages, birth defects, central nervous disorders, epilepsy, urinary tract diseases and horrible skin eruptions that people began calling "hooker bumps" after Hooker Chemical, the company that had done the dumping.

Love Canal, chemical waste dump area

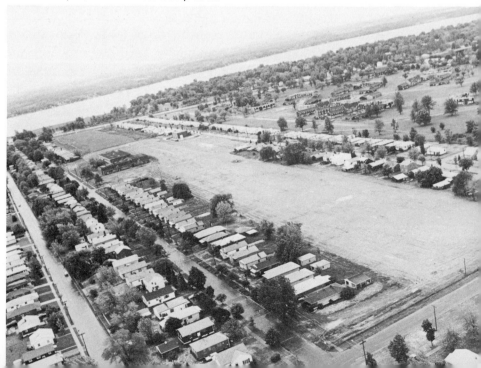

Lois succeeded in getting the school closed down. Together with other women, she went on to organize the Love Canal Home Owners' Association, which sought to force the authorities to do a health study and come up with a solution to this problem they were living with. It took two painful, eye-opening years of work, but finally they got the State of New York and the federal government to admit the awful implications and move the residents out of Love Canal.

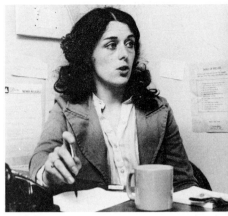

Lois Gibbs

"This is just the beginning. We have not found one third of the illnesses or one third of the damages done," Lois testified before the congressional committee investigating Love Canal. "It is just the tip of the iceberg. We are not the only one. Everyone has one in their backyard somewhere, whether it is hiding or whether it is exposed. We are the first, but we are not likely to be the last. Something must be done," she told them. "I ask that you do what you can for us and do what you *must,* and I emphasize *must,* to prevent what has happened at Love Canal from ever happening again."

There are women like Lois all over the country. Just plain moms who never considered themselves leaders or agitators, but who rise to heights of real courage and determination when their families' health is endangered. Whether the issue is a toxic chemical dump at Love Canal in New York or in Riverside, California; the effects of aerial herbicide spraying of Agent Orange in Oregon in the 1970s or of radioactive fallout in St. George, Utah, from above-ground atomic testing in the 1950s; whether it is a mysterious outbreak of leukemia in Rutherford, New Jersey, or the brown lung disease endemic in cotton mills throughout the South, women are speaking out and mobilizing their communities to do something about it.

Women's Workplaces, Women's Health

Another place where women are beginning to assume responsibility for their well-being is in the office. Lest this seem a parochial concern, bear in mind that clerical workers make up the largest sector of the work force and that women hold 80 percent of these jobs. The Department of Labor predicts that office work will be the fastest growing occupational field in the 1980s with nearly five million new jobs.

Secretaries rank second-highest as victims of stress-related diseases, including heart disease. The Framingham Heart Study found that among women with children and blue-collar husbands, those doing clerical jobs run twice the risk of heart disease as the cross-section of men who participated in the study. And that women doing clerical work, regardless of marital status and family size, suffer twice as much heart disease as other women.

Researchers have identified the main causes of stress among clerical workers as lack of control over their work environment, lack of decision-making responsibility on the job, economic stress (low pay, dead-end jobs), and unsupportive bosses.

An office-work revolution is beginning that could improve the white-collar environment—or make it an even greater health hazard. This is the widespread integration of advanced computer, micro-electronic and telecommunications technology used to process and transmit information. It combines word and data processing and links today's modern devices into "integrated office systems." This may "bring about an organizational revolution among white collar workers," predicts computer specialist James Carlisle, "comparable in magnitude to that resulting from the introduction of the assembly line in blue collar work."

Today's automated office, in fact, resembles more and more an assembly line where workers are expected to perform one function all day long, tiny fractions of the larger task. This requires less training, less initiative and offers less potential for advancement. Office workers are expected to do these tasks at an accelerated pace, which is monitored by computer. Production quotas are increased according to the capacity of the new machine, but additional break time is rarely granted.

The key unit of the new automated office is the VDT, the video display terminal, which processes texts or data and is linked to a computer system. Studies show that VDT typists suffer from extreme fatigue, feelings of alienation, monotony and lack of challenge in their jobs at twice the rate of traditional clerical workers. In fact, a 1979–80 study by The National Institute of Occupational Safety and Health (NIOSH) found that clerical VDT operators showed higher stress ratings than any other group of workers NIOSH has ever studied, including air-traffic controllers!

Recent studies link VDTs to eyestrain, migraine headaches, nausea, lower and upper back pain, depression, high levels of anxiety, digestive problems, short-term loss of visual clarity and temporary changes in color perception.

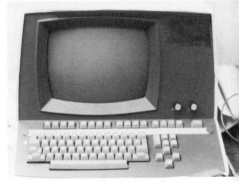

Recent studies link video display terminals to many ailments

A further concern is long-term exposure to low-level radiation from the cathode ray tubes in VDTs. The appearance of eye cataracts in relatively young newspaper VDT operators has been investigated, but not explained. A Newspaper Guild official told Working Women, a national association of office workers, "This whole thing may end up like Three Mile Island; we won't know the damage for another ten to twenty years." The lighting for conventional office work is completely inappropriate for VDTs. They require lower illumination and protection from glare. Many problems result from the bad posture and awkward sitting positions the operator is forced to adopt to compensate for difficulties caused by poor lighting, illegible original copies and poor work-station design.

In addition, there is what has come to be known as the "Tight Building Syndrome." Increasingly airtight buildings, new plastic-based synthetic furnishings, chemical insulation materials, exhaust fumes such as ozone from office machines, faulty ventilation and chemical contaminants in photocopiers and other office equipment have led one scientist for the World Health Organization to say, "There's probably more damage to human health by indoor pollution than by outdoor pollution."

One secretary who works as an insurance policy examiner in Boston has lost the ability to produce tears—she has been diagnosed as having allergic conjunctivitis. At least half of the women in her department have developed eye problems which they believe are related to the irritating fumes from the photocopying machines and other chemicals in a building that lacks proper ventilation. Management states that there is nothing wrong with the air, yet everyone who goes to an ophthalmologist learns the same thing: "It's from the building you work in."

None of the health hazards that now exist in offices is inevitable. Proper ventilation, substituting safe products for those containing toxic substances, properly maintained office equipment, and laws to ensure improved indoor air quality can all be implemented. The new technology

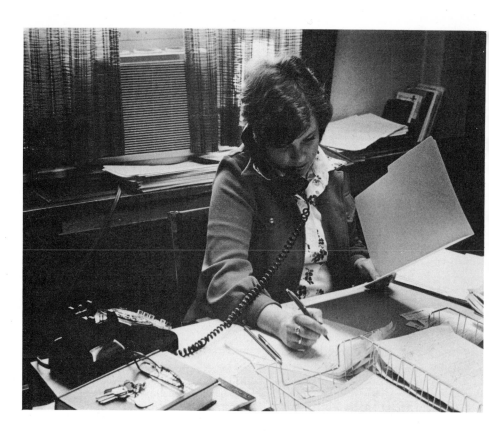

is still in its formative years. The health hazards I have mentioned need not be locked permanently into clerical work.

Clerical workers themselves are beginning to speak out and take the initiative on these issues. They want to feel that the computer is an extension of them, not they an extension of the computer. They know that regular rest breaks are essential, as is the redesign of the jobs to be done. They are demanding that employers institute a system of job rotation to avoid constant sitting and repetition. They also are demanding to be supplied with appropriate chairs, better designed work stations and machines.

The union to which Austrian VDT operators belong has demanded that a person be required to work on the VDT for only an hour at a time and should do traditional office work in between these shifts. The British Postal Service's contract with its employees stipulates that "normal maximum periods at VDTs not exceed 100 minutes a day, and that no operator be required to work more than 50 minutes without a break."

Office work is not the only hazardous on-the-job exposure for women. Nine to five in the office, or three to eleven on the swing shift in the electronics industry, all night long in a hospital laboratory or living-in twenty-four hours a day as a domestic, women experience a variety of dangerous exposures. The table below lists a number of hazardous occupations that employ large numbers of women.

Occupational Exposures in Trades Employing Large Numbers of Women

Occupation	Exposure
Textile and related occupations	
Textile workers	Raw cotton dust, noise, synthetic fiber dusts, formaldehyde, heat, dyes, flame retardants, asbestos
Sewers and stitchers, upholsterers	Cotton and synthetic fiber dusts, noise, formaldehyde, organic solvents, benzene, toluene, trichloroethylene, perchloroethylene, chloroprene, styrene, carbon disulfide, flame retardants, asbestos
Hospital and health personnel	
Registered nurses, aides, orderlies	Anesthetic gases, ethylene oxide, X-ray radiation, alcohol, infectious diseases, puncture wounds
Dental hygienists	X-ray radiation, mercury, ultrasonic noise, anesthetic gases
Laboratory workers (clinical and research)	Wide variety of toxic chemicals, including carcinogens, mutagens, and teratogens, X-ray radiation
Electronics assemblers	Lead, tin, antimony, trichloroethylene, methylene chloride, epoxy resins, methyl ethyl ketone
Hairdressers and cosmetologists	Hair spray resins (polyvinyl pyrrolidone), aerosol propellants (freons), halogenated hydrocarbons, hair dyes, solvents of nail polish, benzyl alcohol, ethyl alcohol, acetone
Cleaning personnel	
Launderers	Soaps, detergents, enzymes, heat, humidity, industrially contaminated clothing
Dry cleaners	Perchloroethylene, trichloroethylene, stoddard solvent (naphtha), benzene, industrially contaminated clothing
Photographic processors	Caustics, iron salts, mercuric chloride, bromides, iodides, pyrogallic acid, silver nitrate
Plastic fabricators	Acrylonitrile, phenol formaldehydes, urea formaldehydes, hexamethylenetetramine, acids, alkalies, peroxide, vinyl chloride, polystyrene, vinylidene chloride
Domestics	Solvents, hydrocarbons, soaps, detergents, bleaches, alkalies
Transportation personnel	Carbon monoxide, polynuclear aromatics, lead, and other combustion products of gasoline, vibration, physical stress
Sign painters and letterers	Lead oxide, lead chromate pigments, epichlorohydrin, titanium dioxide, trace metals, xylene, toluene
Clerical personnel	Physical stress, poor illumination, trichloroethylene, carbon tetrachloride and various other cleaners, asbestos in air conditioning
Opticians and lens grinders	Coal tar pitch volatiles, iron oxide, dust solvents hydrocarbons
Printing personnel	Ink mists, 2-nitropropane, methanol, carbon tetrachloride, methylene chloride, lead, noise, hydrocarbon solvents, trichloroethylene, toluene, benzene, trace metals

Source: U.S. Department of Health, Education, and Welfare, National Institute for Occupational Safety and Health, *Guidelines on Pregnancy and Work* (Washington, D.C.: U.S. Government Printing Office, 1977), pp. 65–66.

Nor should it be forgotten that women whose work is primarily in the home—and indeed all women who do housework—are exposed to the hazards of household products produced by the same industries that bring you all the other perils I have been describing. Vinyl chloride, for instance, a proven cause of liver, lung, and brain cancer, was a spray-can propellant in such items as household insect killers until it was finally banned by the government. It was shown that the use of such sprays for only a few seconds equaled or exceeded the exposure to workers involved in its manufacture.

And it is also true that the stress designed into the work environment is reflected back again and multiplied by the stresses built into our society and economic system as a whole. Lack of control and economic stress on the job have their counterparts in our daily lives where we have no input into corporate decisions that may drastically affect our lives, whether it be through introducing a hazardous product into the marketplace or disposing of toxic wastes into our environment.

Nor does alienation punch out with the time clock. Cirrhosis of the liver, which is one of the ravages of the disease of alcoholism, kills 30,000 Americans every year. Cigarette smoking is a major contributor to lung cancer and heart disease. Drug abuse takes a heavy toll. Perhaps the most serious indictment of our stressful environment is that the leading four causes of death among men and women between fifteen and thirty-four are cancer, accidents, suicides and homicides! More than 60,000 of our young people die violently every year. And this is a time of peace.

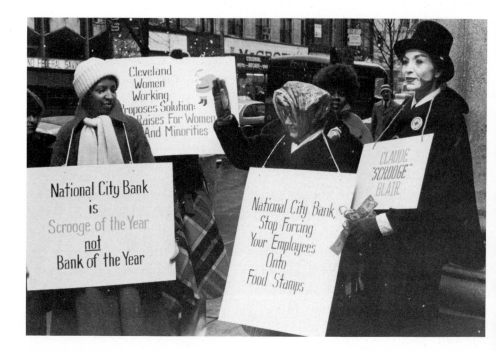

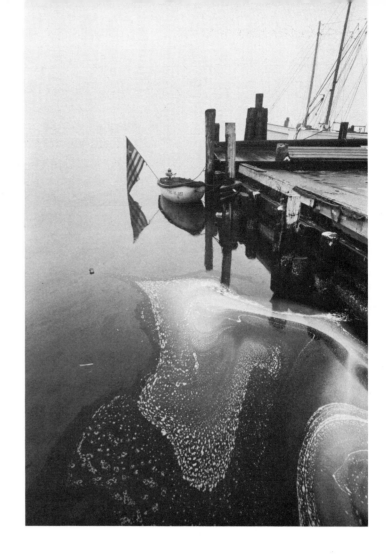

It Is Up to Us

Food that's fit to eat on the table, a schoolyard that's safe for children to play in and a beach where they are not afraid to swim, air that is safe to breathe at work and at home: these used to seem like simple, taken-for-granted things and they should be. Health does *not have* to be sacrificed on the corporate altar of efficiency and profit. Cancer and other diseases are *not* an inevitable by-product of progress.

We do not need to roll back the techno-chemical advances of the last four decades (even if we could). There is no going back. We cannot unlearn what we already know and those who, ostrich-like, advocate doing so are wasting their good intentions.

We can, however, and must, guide the uses to which these technologies are applied. We can ensure that their applications not be irresponsible and shortsighted, that the criteria for their application serve ecological and social ends—not simply economic ones.

It's up to us. As individuals, we can decide not to eat a *"real"* dinner at McDonald's, or Taco Bell's; we can incorporate more natural, healthful foods into our diet; we can exercise daily. But if our private decisions concerning our own health are to have real meaning, we must actively, aggressively and systematically confront the larger questions of our national policy. For it is ultimately those policy decisions that determine how safe our diet, our environment and our workplace will be.

It has never been easy and it will be harder now. The current administration in Washington seems to think that federal regulations designed to protect the environment would be better used to serve the interests of corporate boardrooms. Luella Kenny is a neighbor and friend of Lois Gibbs's at Love Canal. In her appeal for corporate responsibility to Occidental Petroleum (the owners of Hooker Chemical, the company that dumped toxic wastes at Love Canal), Luella said: "We don't have to worry about the luxuries we can't afford because of inflation. And why worry about an enemy who will destroy us, when we are self-destructing? We don't need sophisticated nuclear weapons. All we need are the multitude of dumps strategically placed all over the country that will insidiously destroy everything and everyone in its path." Luella Kenny, like Lois Gibbs, had never spoken out publicly before the crisis at Love Canal. Her voice and others like hers must now be turned toward our political leaders and policy-makers. If they turn a deaf ear, then our voices must be raised until they listen.

It is up to us. No one is going to do it for us.

NOTES

page 20   ". . . such as the wives of Generals Thieu and Ky" Tom Hayden, *The Love of Possession Is a Disease with Them* (New York: Holt, Rinehart and Winston, 1972).

page 33   ". . . than they did on a low-fiber diet of 2,500 calories" Mark Bricklin, *Lose Weight Naturally* (Emmaus, Pa.: Rodale Press, 1979), p. 93.

page 35   ". . . an increase in the amount of sugar we consume" Letitia Brewster and Michael F. Jacobson, Ph.D., *The Changing American Diet* (Washington, D.C.: Center for Science in the Public Interest, 1978), p. 3.

page 37   ". . . close to 90 percent of the beef and poultry raised for market in this country have been on antibiotics and drugs all their lives" Harrison Wellford, *Sowing the Wind* (New York: Bantam Books, 1973), p. 126.

page 40   ". . . research which indicates that what you eat early in the day is less fattening than what you eat at night" Mark Bricklin, *Lose Weight Naturally* (Emmaus, Pa.: Rodale Press, 1979), pp. 213–214.

page 47   ". . . a woman is raped every other minute" Jane E. Brody in *The New York Times*, October 15, 1980.

page 49   ". . . less physical exertion than taking a shower" *President's Association of Physical Fitness Directors in Business and Industry.*

page 50   ". . . one out of every three Americans is overweight" Marie V. Krause and Kathleen L. Mahan, *Food, Nutrition and Diet Therapy* (New York: W. B. Saunders, 1979), p. 556.

page 230   ". . . government and industry's past failure to properly protect our groundwater" *Interim Report on Groundwater Contamination: Environmental Protection Agency Oversight Committee on Government Operations*, 96th Congress, September 1980.

page 231   ". . . he felt air pollution was under 'substantial control' " Article by Jack Nelson entitled "Pollution Curbed, Reagan Says; Attacks Air Cleanup" in the *Los Angeles Times*, October 9, 1980.

page 233   ". . . brings us Ma Brown's pickles" Jim Hightower, *Eat Your Heart Out* (New York: Vintage Books, 1976), p. 21.

page 233   ". . . fifty companies that reap about 70% of the total profits of the food industry" ibid., p. 21.

page 234   ". . . the same quality, price competition, choice and product reliability" ibid., p. 12.

page 234   ". . . we paid at least $16 billion too much for the food we bought in 1980" Arthur E. Rowse, *Help: The Indispensable Almanac of Consumer Information, 1981* (New York: Everest House, 1980), p. 192.

page 234   ". . . three billion dollars is spent on food advertising every year" ibid., p. 191.

page 235   ". . . there is only two cents' worth of wheat in Wheaties" Jim Hightower, *Eat Your Heart Out* (New York: Vintage Books, 1976), pp. 61–62.

page 235   ". . . Wheaties with an extra two cents' worth of synthetic vitamins sprayed on" Dr. Michael F. Jacobson, *Nutrition Scoreboard* (Washington, D.C.: Center For Science in the Public Interest, July 1973), p. 88.

Also see: Jim Hightower, *Eat Your Heart Out* (New York: Vintage Books, 1976), p. 15.

page 236   ". . . these 2500 ingredients react to each other when they come together in the stomach" Jim Hightower, op. cit., p. 106.

page 236   ". . . vital genetic blueprints for all living species" Tom Alexander, "The Hysteria About Food Additives," *Fortune Magazine*, March 1972, p. 64.

page 236   ". . . learning disabilities in some children have been linked to food colorings and flavorings" Ben F. Feingold, M.D., "Are We Becoming Paranoid About Additives In Food?" *Washington Post*, September 19, 1974, p. F-1.

page 237   ". . . More to the point, why should we be dumb enough to let them" Jim Hightower, op. cit., p. 279.

page 238   ". . . This year, it will claim more than 400,000 nationwide" *Cancer Facts and Figures*, American Cancer Society, 1981.

page 239   ". . . very possibly the worst, threat to human health in the nation today" *Health Effects of Toxic Pollution: A Report from the Surgeon General* (Washington, D.C.: U.S. Government Publication, August 1980), p. 153.

page 239   ". . . among the population exposed to asbestos, more than two million will die of cancer" Mark Green, "The Progressive Alternative to Indifference" in *The Village Voice*, March 25–31, 1981, p. 14.

page 239   ". . . and most of them have not been tested for carcinogenic effects" Testimony by Dr. Samuel Epstein, Professor of Occupational and Environmental Medicine, School of Public Health, Univ. of Illinois, to the California State Hearing on Toxic Waste Management, November 1980.

page 240   ". . . calls the dumps 'toxic time bombs' " ibid.

page 240   ". . . but very little of that money went to prevention" Samuel S. Epstein, M.D., *The Politics of Cancer* (New York: Anchor/Doubleday, 1979), p. 331.

page 244   ". . . suffer twice as much heart disease as other women" Dept. of Health, Education & Welfare, *Proceedings of Conference on Occupational Stress* (Cincinnati, Ohio: NIOSH Publication, March 1978), pp. 78–156.

Also see: Working Women, *Race Against Time* (Cleveland, Ohio: National Association of Office Workers, April 1980), for results of Framingham Heart Study.

page 244   ". . . the introduction of the assembly line in blue collar work" As quoted in John Markoff and John Stewart, "The Microprocessor Revolution: An Office on the Head of a Pin," *In These Times*, March 3-17, 1979.

page 245   ". . . monotony and lack of challenge in their jobs" A. Cakir, with D. J. Hart and T. F. M. Stewart, *The VDT Manual* (Darmstadt, Germany: 1979) See Chapter 5: "The Health, Safety & Organizational Aspects of Working With VDTs." See also Gunilla Bradley, *Computerization and Psychosocial Factors in the Working Environment* (Institute of Sociology, University of Stockholm).

page 245   ". . . including air-traffic controllers." U.S. Dept. of Health and Human Services, NIOSH, *Health Consequences of Video Viewing: San Francisco Study* February 1981. See also Michael J. Smith, Ph.D., et al., *VDTs: A Preliminary Health Risk Evaluation*, NIOSH, January 1980.

page 245 ". . . short-term loss of visual clarity" NIOSH, op. cit.

Also see: Smith, op. cit.

page 245 ". . . poor lighting, illegible original copies and poor work-station design" National Association of Office Workers, *Race Against Time: Automation of the Office,* report by Working Women Education Fund (Cleveland, Ohio, 1980).

page 245 ". . . more damage to human health by indoor pollution than by outdoor pollution" *Warning: Health Hazards for Office Workers, An Overview of Problems and Solutions in Occupational Health in the Office.* Report by Working Women Education Fund (Cleveland, Ohio, April 1981), p. 29.

page 245 ". . . it's from the building you work in" ibid., p. 30.

page 246 ". . . that no operator be required to work more than 50 minutes without a break" *Testimony of Andrea Hricko, L.O.H.P. Before the State of California's Industrial Welfare Commissions, Wage Board #4, Concerning the Need for Rest Breaks for VDT Users,* April 12, 1979.

page 250 ". . . that will insidiously destroy everything and everyone in its path" *Statement to the Annual Meeting of Occidental Petroleum Shareholders, Corporate Responsibility Resolution,* May 21, 1980.

PHOTO CREDITS